Yoga *for*
Sex

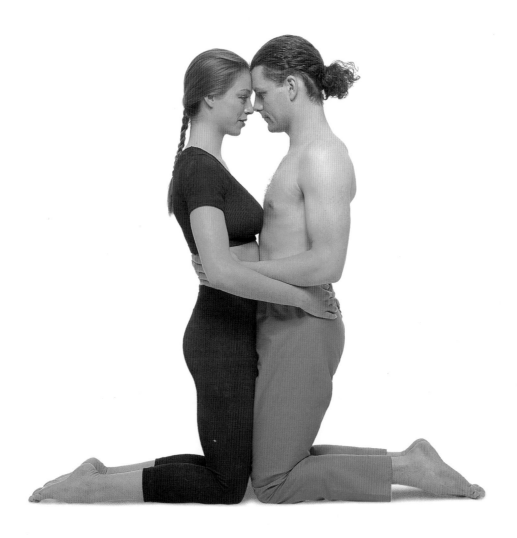

Yoga *for* Sex

Vimla Lalvani

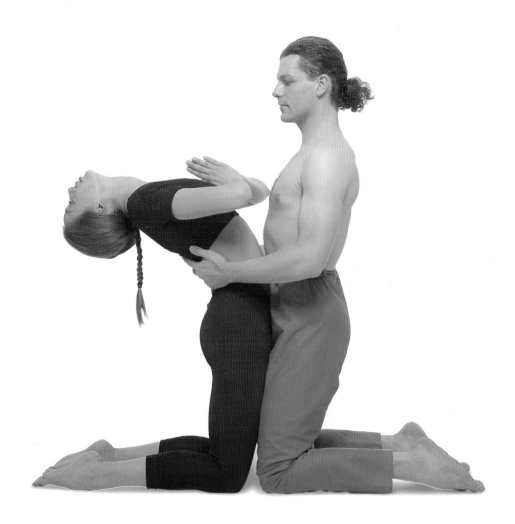

HAMLYN

Contents

First published in Great Britain in 1997 by Hamlyn, an imprint of
Octopus Publishing Group Limited
2-4 Heron Quays, London E14 4JP
Text © The Natural Therapy Company Limited 1997
Design © Octopus Publishing Group Limited 1997
Photographs © Octopus Publishing Group Limited 1997
Reprinted 1999

The moral right of the author has been asserted

ISBN 0 600 59243 X

A CIP catalogue record for this book is available from the British Library.

Printed and bound in Hong Kong

SAFETY NOTE: It is advisable to check with your doctor before embarking on any exercise program. While the advice and information in this book are believed to be accurate and the step-by-step instructions have been devised to avoid strain, neither the author nor the publisher can accept any legal responsibility for any injury sustained while following the exercises. With the prevalence of AIDS and other sexually transmitted diseases, if you do not practise safe sex you are risking your life and your partner's life.

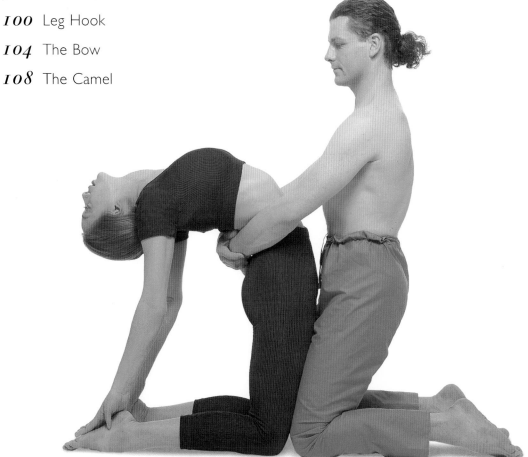

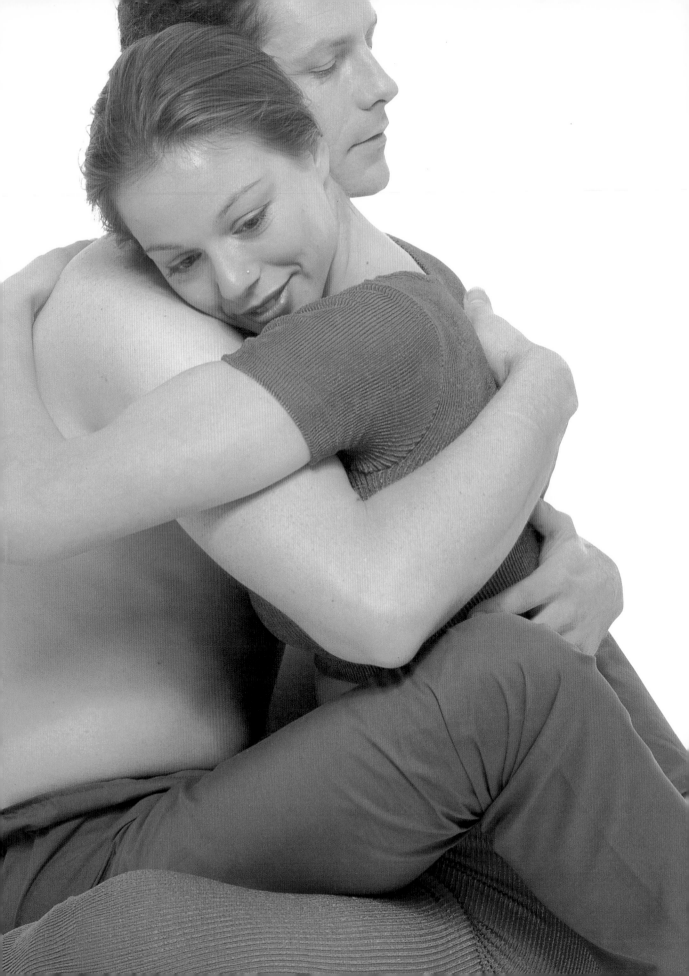

Introduction
Better sex with yoga

There is no more important sexual organ in the human body than the mind, no physical or mental experience or sensation-complex more ecstatic and blissful than an ideal and complete sexual union between two truly loving partners. However, when the mind, body and soul are not integrated there is a great deal of unhappiness; feelings of frustration and negative thoughts result, in turn leading to irrational and inappropriate behavior. If one partner in a sexual relationship feels inadequate and incapable of giving pleasure to the other, there is a loss of self-worth and the relationship usually degenerates. Ignorance, anxiety and fear regarding the quality and effectiveness of one's sexual performance dampens the ardor between even the most loving couples.

Sexual compatibility is an integral part of every relationship and when frustration and disharmony set in there is a breakdown in every level of the relationship. Yoga teaches you how to channel your energy in a positive manner as well as giving you techniques to better your sex life; it is a natural aphrodisiac and sexual conditioner that unites the mind, body, and soul.

In Sanskrit, *yug* is the root word of *yoga*, which means to unite. In Hatha yoga, the union of mind and body is described through physical exercises, or asanas, to harmonize and balance the masculine and feminine energies that exist equally in both men and women; in Tantric yoga, harmony and balance are achieved through the sexual union between a man and woman.

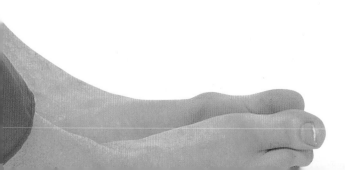

Yoga philosophy states that there are different paths to a spiritual union with God, and mystics, religious leaders, and Indian sages often speak of divine ecstasy in this context. The rituals of prayer and techniques that require intense discipline lead to this path. This divine ecstasy is also often described when sexual orgasm is total and complete, and some people equate this sensation with divine bliss.

Though not everyone shares a spiritual goal, everyone can experience the improvement that yoga brings to one's life, including its sexual dimension. Yoga provides a natural solution for anyone seeking harmony and balance as it teaches techniques that help discipline the mind and body and explains how to take control of sexual passions rather than being ruled by them.

Not only does yoga promote a calm nervous system, it gives you the suppleness and flexibility that are required in lovemaking and also teaches you how to breathe correctly, bringing extra vitality and energy to the sexual act. By bending and twisting in various positions you will stimulate the internal organs and send fresh oxygen to the blood flow, thus rejuvenating and regenerating the cells. The immune system is boosted and the result is an invigorated body and an inner calm with a positive mental attitude.

The exercises in this book are designed to improve your sexual performance by increasing your stamina and your ability to stretch. The movements are graceful and fluid, like a dancer's, and are held for a length of time in order to allow the body's energy to alter. The yogic and sexual exercises both have the same goal; when they are intelligently and properly performed they will lead to longevity, alertness, radiant health, contentment, serenity, and tranquility. Both yoga and sexual satisfaction promote tolerance and forgiveness, enrich the emotional life, and illuminate the concept of truth and beauty.

Yoga is not a religion, but a philosophy of life. It has a universal appeal and does not interfere with anyone's belief system; it has a scientific base and in order to enjoy its benefits you do not need to have faith in it – it is enough simply to practise it. The person having no faith in yoga as a philosophy will receive exactly the same benefits through its practice as the ardent believer.

Yoga elevates and spiritualizes sex itself, the added ecstasy of the spirituality of yoga adding to the physical thrill of sex. The orgasmic explosion is intensified and post-coital tranquility takes on an element of the divine. The facts of sex are consistent from person to person, race to race, and country to country, although conventions and customs may vary tremendously between one culture and another. However, even though the concept of morality also varies within different cultures, yoga philosophy focuses on the concept of universal love and the relationship that exists between a truly loving couple. It does not advocate promiscuity or homosexuality but considers the perfect union between a man and woman as sacred. It is this union that transcends all cultural boundaries, all religious dogmas, all reason and intelligence to enter into the realms of spiritual truth and divine bliss.

Good sex and bad sex

Most people have had experience of both good sex and bad sex, and know the vast differences in sensation that can be aroused by what is essentially the same physical act. Bad sex leads to dissatisfaction and frustration, making you bad-tempered and difficult to deal with, while good sex creates deep satisfaction, calming and steadying the mind. With good sex there comes a cultural and spiritual refinement, especially when yoga is included as a part of a daily regime. Therefore, a proper exercise of a healthy sex urge combined with yoga's scientific approach will give you a sense of the sublime that will fill your entire mind, body, and spirit.

The practice of yoga tends to resolve the emotional and psychological conflicts that affect sexual performance and at the same time integrates harmoniously the working of the nervous system at the brain and spinal cord levels. The sexual act is controlled by three sections of the nervous system. The first is the somatic nervous system, which deals with reception and perception of the senses of smell, touch, sight, and hearing. This system controls the higher sensory functions of the brain which play such an important role in sexual attraction and behavior. The second system integral to sexual response is the spinal cord, which controls spontaneous reactions, reflecting the primordial sexual drive.

Finally, the third section is the autonomic nervous system. This is an involuntary system which functions on an unconscious level, controlling certain organs, blood vessels and glands as well as hormonal secretions. Its function is to integrate harmoniously the sympathetic and parasympathetic nervous systems, which are naturally antagonistic but need to be well coordinated for the sexual act to be satisfactory. The nerves which control the parasympathetic nervous system are located in the lower part of the spinal cord and are responsible for the erection of the penis and clitoris. It is the sympathetic nervous system that is responsible for the contraction of the seminal vesicles and therefore the ejaculation of semen.

The vast majority of sexual problems are caused by emotional and psychological conflicts rather than by any physical shortcomings afflicting either or both partners. Tranquility of the nervous system is evident in those who practise yoga, and once harmony is achieved within and between the three sections of the nervous system mentioned above, volition control can be achieved through the practice of Tantric sex.

Tantric sex

Tantric yoga is the philosophy of reaching the goal of spiritual enlightenment through sexual techniques, while Tantric sex is the system of rituals, sexual practices, visualization, and meditation that will aid in reaching this goal. In the body there are seven important chakras, or energy centers, and it is vital that each is unblocked of negative energy. Each chakra is a wheel of energy that radiates through the vital centers of the spine. These chakras pick up cosmic vibrations like radio antennae pick up sound waves and distribute them evenly throughout the energy centers. Each center corresponds to the physical body and sometimes emotional disturbances will block the flow of energy, causing an imbalance to the nervous system.

The first chakra is within the pelvic region and corresponds to sexual energy. It is called the base chakra and is the most powerful and important one because it creates life. If this energy is blocked it will create a high-tension area until it explodes, usually in a violent manner. If on the other hand this center is excited, causing the energy to unwind and rise up, it will recharge all the other chakras until it forces its powerful energy through the crown chakra at the top of the head. During sexual intercourse the pumping of energy in the base chakra is a necessary ingredient to fulfilling sex. Those who have an active center will reach a climax extremely quickly, while those with a sluggish center will have difficulty in achieving a climax at all.

Tantric sex teaches techniques to heighten the sexual act by controlling the pace of vibrations. One of these techniques is to refrain from physical contact and subtly raise the base energy together. Vibrations are a powerful force and sometimes people experience a feeling of going weak at the knees at a mere glance from another person. Refraining from the sex act arouses desire, especially when sexual attraction is strong. Sex is only one form of exchanging energy and when visualization and meditation are used also to exchange this energy a mystical climax is achieved even though no physical contact has occurred. Alternatively, this technique can be used as foreplay to the physical act. When desire is so heightened, physical touch stimulates the senses to such a degree as to create an ultimate orgasm of physical pleasure.

The *Kama Sutra*

The *Kama Sutra*, written by the great sage Vatsyayana, is an ancient text from the Vedas that describes the science and art of lovemaking. Historically, it is the same era that gave us Pantajali's Yoga Sutras, ancient writings that describe and explain the significance of yoga. In Hinduism, sex is almost sacramental; it is considered essential to life and worthy of serious study. Vatsyayana said that pleasures are necessary for the well-being of the body, and the Kama asanas, or love poses, enhance pleasure beyond normal expectations. These poses, from the simplest to the most complicated, bear an analogy to classic yoga poses.

When these texts were written over 2000 years ago it was the religious duty of a family man to bear a son to perpetuate the line, and when this was achieved the gates of heaven were opened and the family was truly blessed. All religious leaders during this time gave full attention to the worldly happiness of their people and sexual efficiency was held to be not merely a fundamental right but also a necessary part of the education and culture of the ordinary person, who was expected to be fully conversant in the art and science of love and sex.

Setting the mood

There is so much emphasis today on the pursuit of pleasure, specifically of a sexual nature; we are bombarded by sexual references in advertisements, films, pop music, newspapers, and books. It is a common belief in our society that intoxicants heighten sexual desire and there is a widespread usage of drugs for this purpose, both legally available ones (including alcohol) and banned substances. The people who use these drugs believe that they will arouse and intensify the sex urge. Instead, they dull the senses and neutralize the inhibitions by doping the individual and preventing the sexual sensation experience. Very often, sex loses its importance altogether; the euphoria or hallucination induced by the drugs becomes itself the sole objective.

Within the sex act, intoxicants only affect the brain and its influence upon the spinal centers. The spinal cord itself is not affected, so the sex act becomes a similar experience to that engaged in by an animal and is merely a reflex and instinctive physical action. In reality, there is no aphrodisiac greater than a sexual partner who is the personification of the physical and mental qualities to which you react with warmth, love, desire, and passion; the best means of stimulating your desire is to make love with an exhilarating sexual partner, not to resort to arousal from an artificial chemical compound. When the desired sense-objects give great pleasure even if singly experienced by the senses (soft touch, beautiful sight, entrancing musical sounds, sweet fragrance, and delicious taste), together with the combination of attraction (appearance, age, speech, gestures, actions) real sexual pleasure can be achieved.

What is significantly lacking in modern culture is a clear understanding that even though recreational sex is an important aspect of our lives, certainly in adding greater happiness, a balanced attitude towards sex is equally important. The knowledge and wisdom from the ancient Eastern sages will assist with finding that balance and harmony between the physical and the spiritual that everyone craves.

Yoga integrates the psyche and the benefits are real and lasting. It builds up the philosophical outlook on life, so that the passage of years do not lead to fear, helplessness, impotency, or decrepit old age, but to pleasant, serene, mellow, and mature wisdom. Even in advanced years, health seems to radiate from all parts of the body, including the sex centers.

The sex act should be a spontaneous reflection of one's mood and emotional feeling, but there are nevertheless certain factors that enhance the quality of lovemaking. Setting the mood with music and lighting can contribute to the effect, as can creating an intimate, sensual experience with delicious food and wine. Some people break free of their normal inhibitions by making love in new or unfamiliar surroundings such as on a beach, in a garden, or even just in a different room other than the bedroom. The most important element is to be totally relaxed and have total trust in your partner.

It is naturally more considerate and decent to give your partner the feeling that your love constitutes a total spiritual and emotional response to his or her personality as a whole. Your partner must never feel that your interest in him or her begins and ends with the sex act. The spiritual must be coordinated with the sexual in a truly satisfactory relationship. Certainly, the variety of love poses described in this book will keep the sexual spark alive with vivid imagination and, combined with true love and devotion, will lead you to divine bliss.

How to use this book

I have divided this book into three separate sections. Section 1,
Toning Your Body, concentrates on the self and the individual
need to prepare the physical body for lovemaking and also to
integrate the mind to create inner calm. The exercises in this
section help in building individual strength and stamina while
increasing suppleness and flexibility. The breathing technique will
harmonize your masculine and feminine energies.

Section 2, Prelude, involves a loving couple preparing together
and assisting one another for the poses of the *Kama Sutra*. To be
able to complete the sex act satisfactorily and with complete joy
it is vital that the body be fit enough to withstand the demands
of the physical activity and that the mind be free of worries.
These exercises are designed to equalize each other's
energy and to get in tune with one another through
slow, flowing movements. It can also be used as
foreplay to Section 3, Love Poses.

This last section consists of classical love poses
taken from the ancient *Kama Sutra* text and
teaches you step by step how to achieve the final
poses safely. It describes in detail the physical act and
demystifies these sensual love poses. They become
totally achievable for the average person so
that everyone can experience the
exhilarating pleasure of fulfilling love.

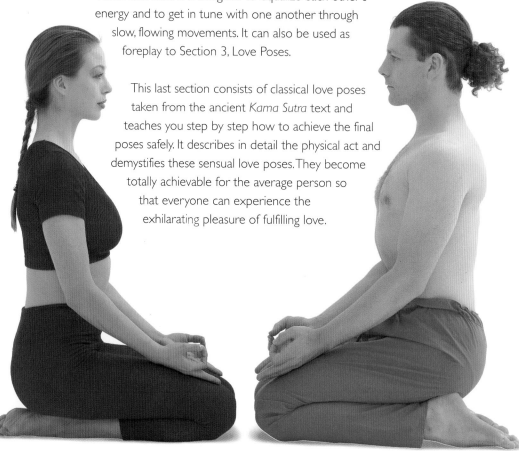

Safety guidelines

There are some important guidelines that must always be followed in order to make sure that you are able to gain all the benefits that yoga has to offer you and that you do not injure yourself while adopting any of the poses in this book.

• These exercises are designed for people who are in a normal state of health. As is the case with any physical exercise program, if you feel unfit or unwell or are recovering from any injury, or if you are pregnant, have high blood pressure or suffer from any medical disorder, you must consult your doctor before embarking upon any of these exercises.

• It is important to follow the instructions in the exercises and to read through each exercise before embarking upon it.

• Never rush the movements and follow the directions exactly. Do not jerk your body and stop immediately if you experience any sharp pain or strain. Never push yourself and always do the pose only to your own capability.

• Pay particular attention to your breathing in order to help relax and focus your mind. Let your deep breathing also relax your body and allow the stretched muscles and ligaments carry more energy to the muscle fibers. Pay attention to your posture, too, and make sure that you always stand, sit or kneel upright.

• When you are in a standing pose you will often be required to balance upon one leg. Keep the leg on which you are standing straight by lifting the muscle above the kneecap. Do not hyper-extend or lock the knee as this can cause injury.

• Choose a warm, quiet, well-ventilated place in which to embark upon any yoga exercises. Make sure you exercise on an even, non-slip surface.

• Do not attempt yoga exercises on a full stomach – allow an interval of one hour after a light meal and four hours after a heavy meal.

• Always follow the recommended warm-up before attempting the main exercises. You can loosen up your muscles even more by taking a shower first.

• Whenever you practise yoga, remember these basic principles: soul/mind control of movements; awareness of postures and movements; slow and deliberate movements; relaxation during movements; go only as far as is comfortable.

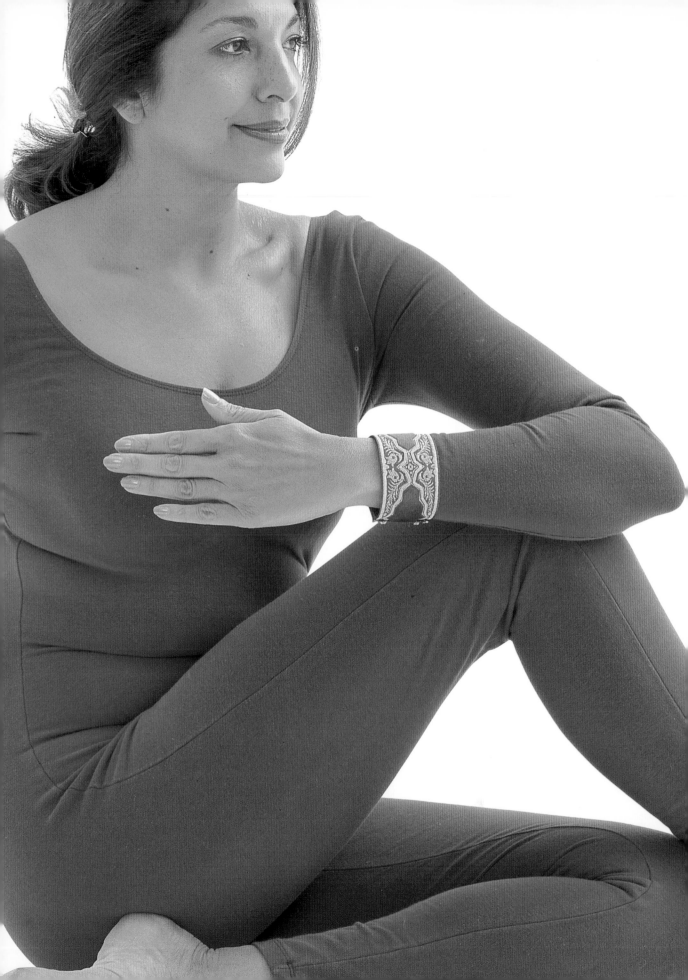

Toning Your Body

These exercises are designed to build muscle tone and stamina and to increase your energy and vitality. When you stretch and twist in all directions you tone your internal organs and, combining that with correct breathing, you send fresh oxygen to each nerve and cell, rejuvenating the entire system. The sex center is located in the lower spine and by strengthening the lower back you will automatically improve your sexual performance.

There is much emphasis today on sexual accomplishment and this is one area where money, status, fame, authority, success, physical strength, and beauty are unable to play a decisive role. These factors may offer a wider choice of partners, but they cannot guarantee a good sexual performance – and unfortunately the stresses and strains which attend many of them actually contribute to sexual disorders.

Confidence and sound mental health remain the greatest assets in the successful consummation of the sex act. Frigidity and fear of coitus in women and lack of an erection or premature ejaculation in men are, in most cases, psychological in origin. The regular practice of yogic exercises will result in not only toning the neuro-muscular structure of the sex organs of both men and women but will rehabilitate the mind as well. Sexual performance will improve when the mind, body, and soul are integrated and the sexual partners are in total harmony with their environment.

Warm Up

Before you begin any yoga exercises it is always important to warm up the body with gentle, easy movements that will reawaken the spine.

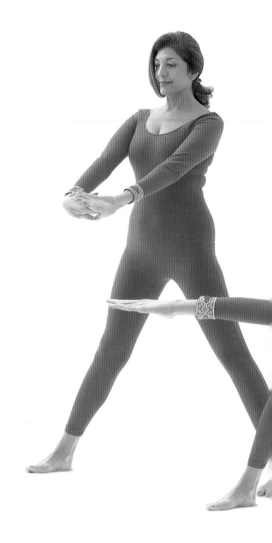

Begin by standing tall in perfect posture, making sure your feet are firmly placed together with your weight evenly distributed between your toes and heels, your shoulders down and your tailbone tucked under. Think of every muscle in your body and tighten and pull in your stomach and buttocks. Imagine that you are growing taller and taller and that there is a piece of string pulling you up from the top of your head. Breathe deeply and slowly from the diaphragm and fill your lungs with fresh oxygen. Center your attention to your breathing pattern and immediately you will feel an inner peace. Deep breathing acts as a natural tranquilizer; the deeper you breathe the calmer the mind becomes. ▸ Place your feet approximately 90cm–1.2m (2–3 ft) apart with your toes pointing forward. Clasp your hands in front of you. ▸ Inhale deeply and stretch your arms over your head. Look up at your hands and drop your head slightly back. ▸ Release your arms and take them behind the small of your back for support. Exhale and slowly drop your head back as far as possible. Push your hips forward and open your throat and chest. Breathe normally and hold for 5 seconds. Return to standing position. ▸ Inhale and stretch your entire body to the left side with your right arm close to your ear, palm facing down. Exhale and place your left arm down on your left leg towards the ankle. As you inhale and exhale deeply try to stretch even further and inch your fingertips down to your feet. ▸ Hold for at least 5 seconds. Repeat the side stretch to the other side, then move on to the warm-up exercise on pages 20–21.

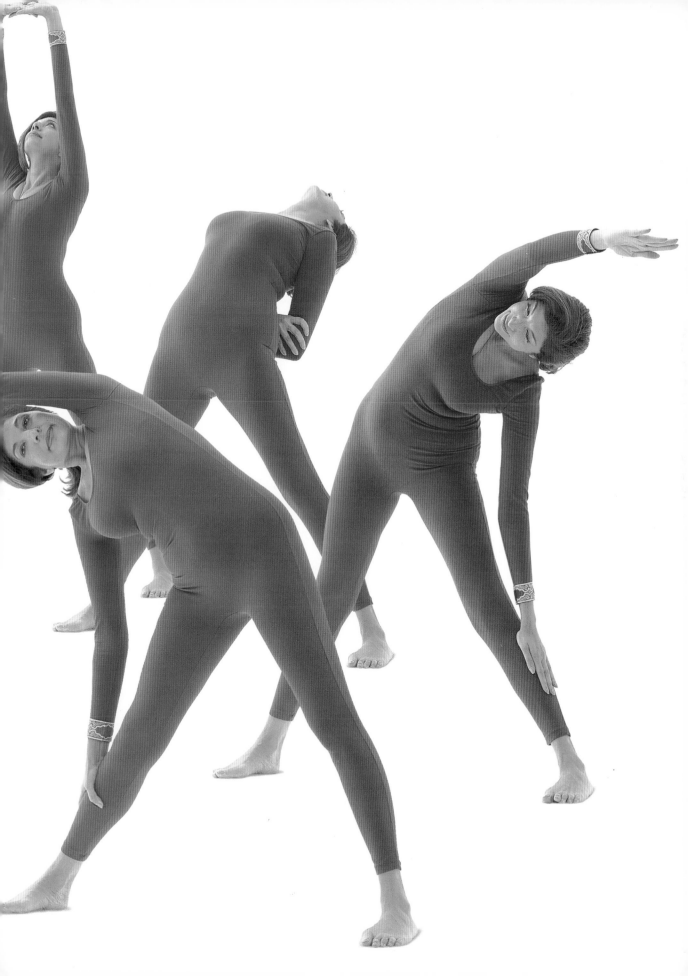

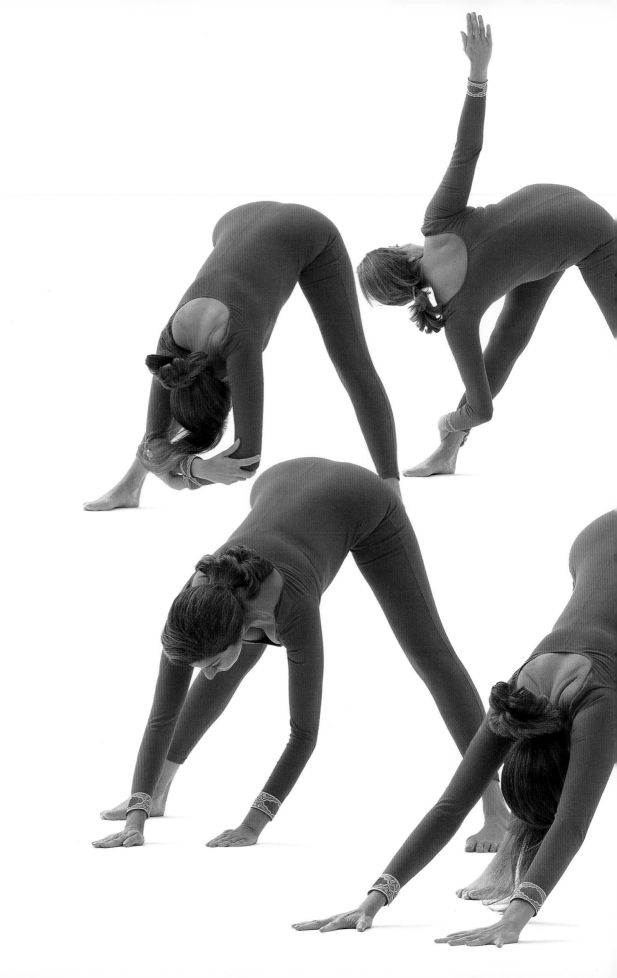

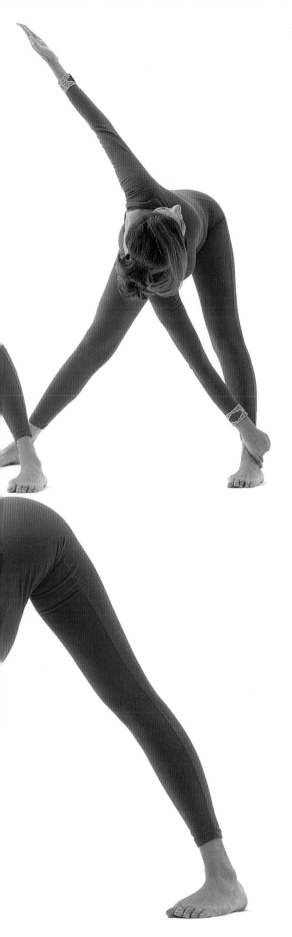

Warm Up
(continued)

Breathe normally, take hold of your left ankle with your right hand and twist your spine, looking over your left shoulder. Keep your left arm straight with your fingertips together. Hold for 5 seconds and slowly increase the stretch. ▶ Change sides, taking your left hand to your right ankle and twisting to look over your right shoulder. Hold for 5 seconds. ▶ Release the twist by holding on to your elbows and hanging forward. Inhale, pull your stomach muscles in, and lift your elbows up as far over your head as possible so your spine is straight. Exhale, breathe normally and hold for 5 seconds. ▶ Release your arms and slowly walk your hands forward as far as possible without moving your feet. ▶ Inhale. Pull your stomach in, exhale, and push your hips back towards your legs, extending your elbows and stretching your spine as much as possible. Breathe deeply and hold for 10 seconds. Relax your back and slowly uncurl your spine until you reach perfect posture.

Balance

This balance combined with deep stretches will help focus your attention and steady your mind. Stretching is the best way to release tension in the muscle groups and this series of movements will increase suppleness and flexibility as well as building muscletone.

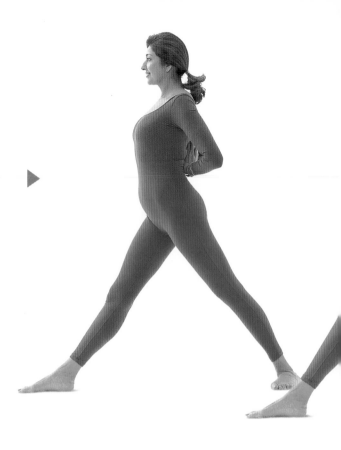

Start the exercise in a wide second position as you did in the Warm Up on page 18. ▶ Turn your right foot to the right with your heel in line with the instep of your left foot. Take your arms behind your back with your palms facing together in a prayer position. This will automatically open the chest. Make sure your shoulders are down and your chin and head level. If you are unable to stretch your arms behind your upper back, hold onto your wrists and place them at your lower back. ▶ Inhale and drop your head back as far as possible. Relax your face and neck. ▶ Exhale and slowly lower your spine, stretching out from the waist, until your forehead touches your knee. Keep your left leg straight and pull up the muscle above your kneecap to help you maintain your balance. ▶ Keep your weight evenly distributed between both feet. Breathing normally, bend your right knee, keeping your head down to the knee. Make sure the back of your knee is directly above your heel. ▶ Release your arms from behind your back and place your right hand down to the floor in line with your shoulder to steady your balance. Fix one point on the floor and concentrate your gaze. Take your left hand to your waist. ▶ Inhale, straighten your right leg and at the same time lift your left leg up so your spine is in a straight line. Flex your left foot. Exhale and hold this position for 10 seconds. To release, return to position 5 and slowly return to the starting position with arms at your sides. Repeat the entire exercise on the other side.

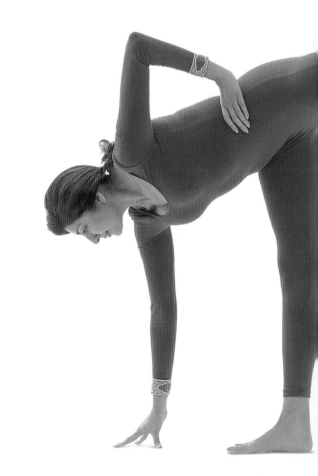

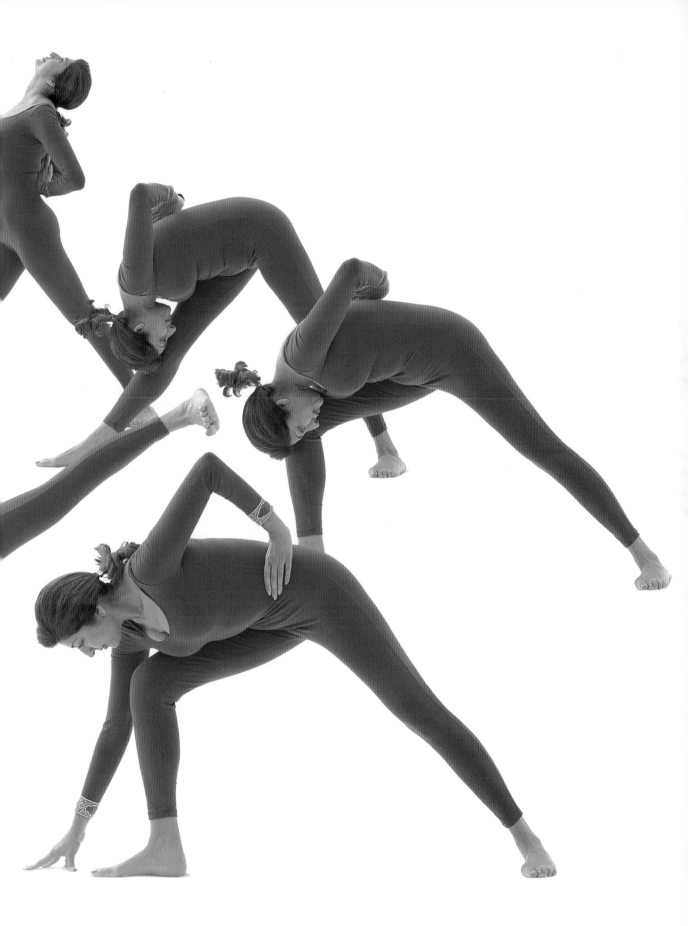

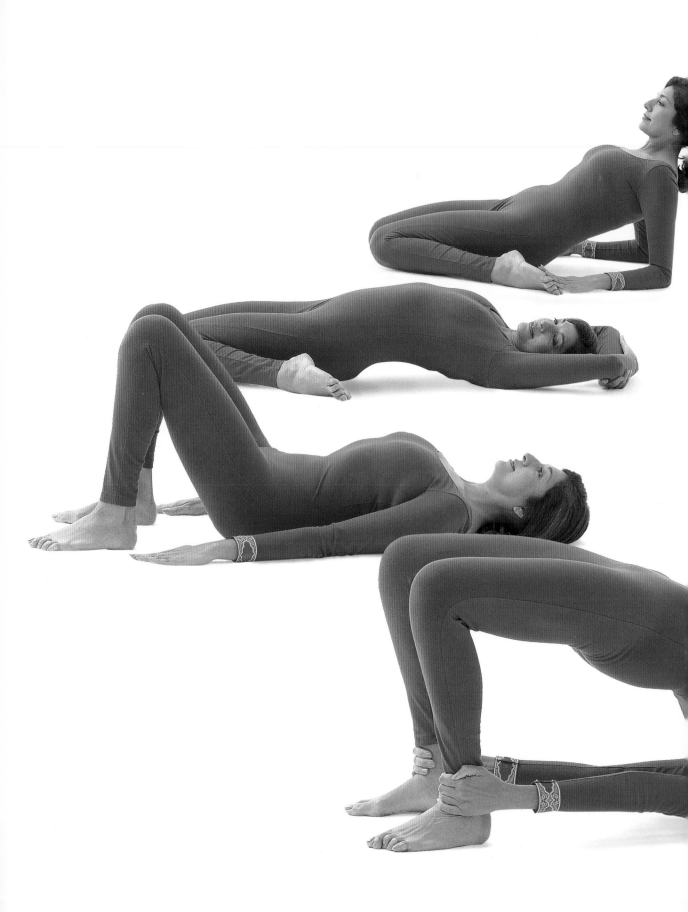

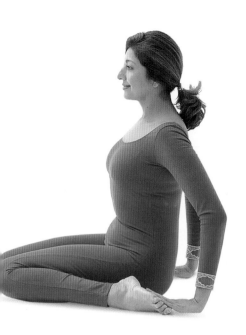

Pelvic Stretch

The pelvic stretch tones the sex organs and the kidneys, aids digestion and rejuvenates the spine. After childbirth or with advancing age, many women suffer from incontinence, a lack of tightness in the vaginal wall and a loss of sensation during sexual intercourse. Learning how to isolate and contract the pelvic muscle will greatly improve these conditions.

Kneel down on the floor, spreading your feet as far apart as you can while keeping your knees together. Place your hands behind you and sit erect. Breathe deeply and evenly. ▶ Keeping your knees together, slowly lower yourself, leaning on your elbows. You will feel a stretch in the feet, ankles, knees, thighs, abdomen, and ribs. If you feel comfortable, stretch further down to the floor, taking your arms over your head holding your elbows. As you breathe deeply and especially during the exhalation you will feel a deep stretching sensation throughout your whole body. This intense stretch sends a fresh blood supply to the entire system and the effect is soothing, tranquil, and deeply relaxing. ▶ To release yourself from this position return to position 2, then 1. Now relax down to the floor with your arms to the side, palms facing down. Raise your knees with your feet in line with your hips. ▶ Inhale, hold onto your ankles, and raise your pelvis as high as possible. Exhale, breathe normally, tighten your stomach and buttock muscles and contract the muscles in the sex centers. Hold for 10 seconds and slowly lower to the floor by pushing down each vertebra of the spine, starting from the neck. Repeat the entire exercise, then move on to the exercises on pages 26–27.

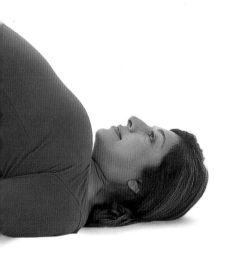

Pelvic Stretch (continued)

Lying on the floor, bring your knees into your chest. Cross your ankles and hold onto your feet. ▶ Inhale, and take your knees down to the floor. Exhale, and hold for 5 seconds, breathing normally. ▶ Inhale, and push up your chest until the top of your head is on the floor. In classic yoga, this pose is called the Fish; it helps corrects certain defects of the spine and sends fresh oxygen and blood supply to the brain, which soothes the nerves. Exhale, breathe normally and lower your back to the floor to return to the previous position. Repeat the exercise. ▶ Now release the legs and lie flat on the floor. Inhale, point both feet and raise the left leg up off the floor toward your head, then raise your upper body off the floor toward the leg. Lift your right leg 30cm (12in) off the floor. Exhale, breathe normally and hold for 5 seconds. Slowly lower your back down to the floor and lift both legs in a right angle to the body. Breathe deeply and hold for 10 seconds. Inhale, lift your body up and hold onto your right ankle, stretching your head to your right knee. Exhale and lower your left leg down to 30cm (12in) from the floor. Point both feet, breathe deeply and hold for 5 seconds. Raise your left leg until both legs are in a 90-degree angle to the floor. Bend both knees into the chest. Inhale, and as you exhale slowly lower the legs down to the floor. Relax for 10 seconds.

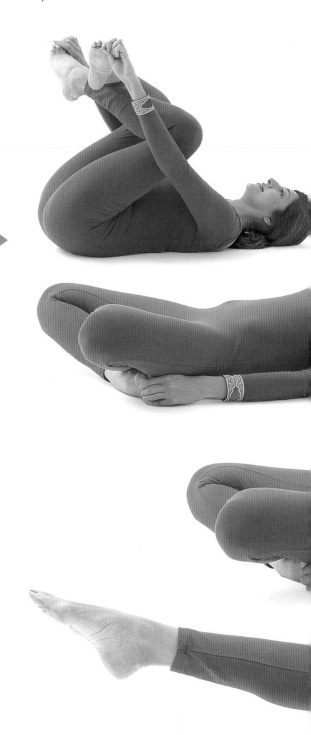

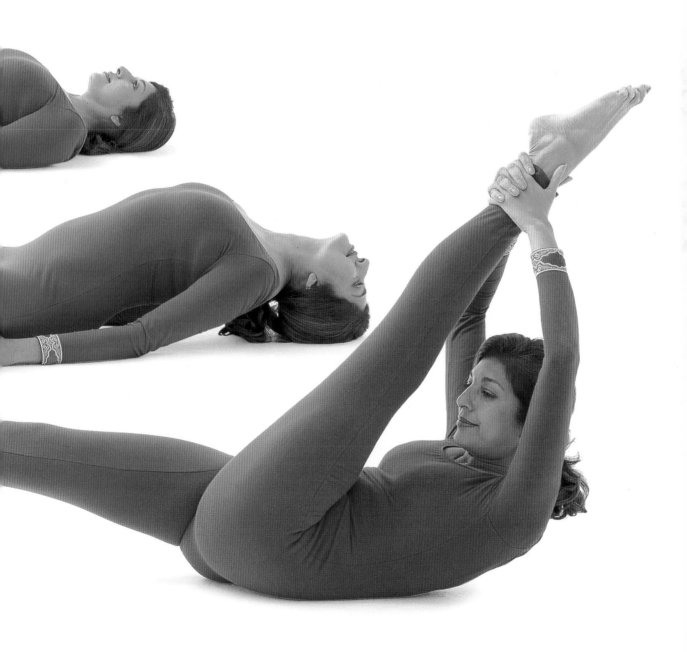

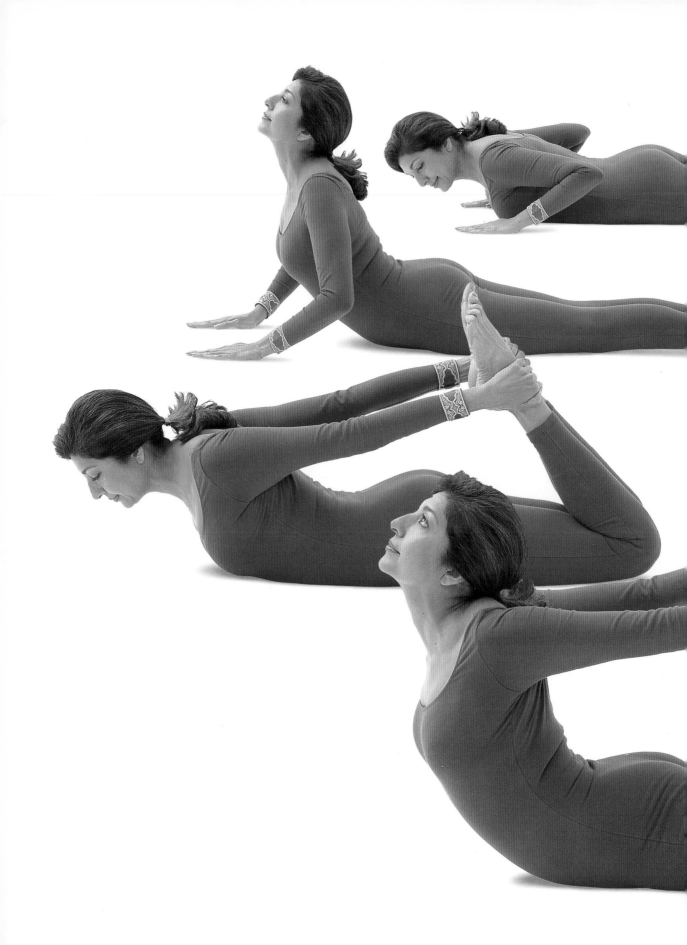

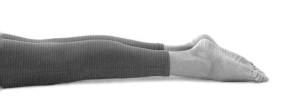

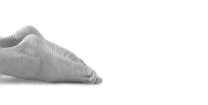

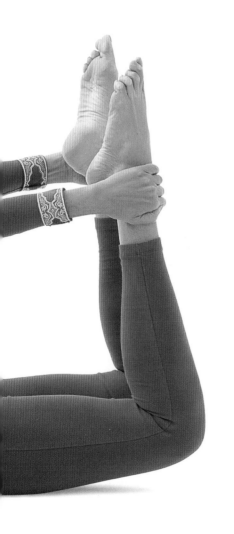

Cobra and Bow

These exercises keep the spine young and flexible even during old age, alleviating back pain and strengthening the lumbar region. They tone up the sex centers in the spine and pelvic organs as well as stimulating the sensory nerves. The pressure placed on the pelvic region during the exercises increases the blood supply to the region, improving the tissues connected to the sexual and urogenital functions. The exercises also dissolve fat from the knees, thighs, hips, waist, and abdomen, improve the circulation to the large intestine, help to eliminate toxins, and neutralize the gastric juices in the digestive process.

Begin by lying flat on your stomach. Place your hands directly under your shoulder blades close to your chest. Make sure your fingertips are pointed forward and your toes are pointed. Lift your head slightly off the floor. ▶ Inhale, push your palms down and lift your spine up as far as possible, keeping your hipbones on the floor. Exhale, breathe normally and hold for 10 seconds. On the exhalation slowly lower your body to the floor. Repeat the exercise and lie back down on the floor. ▶ Take hold of your ankles and with a deep inhalation lift your body and legs up in a shape of a bow .Exhale, breathe deeply and hold for 10 seconds. ▶ As you hold keep stretching upward and try to keep your head in line with your feet. Exhale, release the legs and return to the floor. Repeat the exercise. This is quite a strenuous exercise so when you finish relax down to the floor. Turn your head to one side and wait until your breathing returns to normal.

Sitting Stretch

This yoga stretch improves the tone of the circulatory and neuro-muscular systems of the entire pelvis. It helps to cure menstrual cramps and strengthens the muscles and ligaments of the calves, thighs, and all the joints of the legs. The Sitting Stretch tones up the sex centers and improves the sexual efficiency of the couple – yogis prescribe it to help cure semen defects in men and improve functioning of the ovaries and Fallopian tubes in women.

Begin by sitting up tall with your legs stretched wide apart. Flex your feet and try to push your knees down to the floor, rotating them outward to eliminate any space between them and the floor.
▶ Inhale and reach your right hand round the bottom of your right foot. Place your left hand on your waist. ▶ Bend your right elbow, exhale, and take your left arm over your head close to your ear. Stretch to the right as much as possible. Keep your fingertips together with your palm facing down. Breathe deeply and hold for 10 seconds. Release, return to an upright position and repeat the stretch to the opposite side. Return to an upright position.
▶ Bend forward to take hold of both feet. Inhale, and stretch forward from your waist until your head touches the floor. Never force or jerk your body. Breathe as deeply as possible and you will find your body stretching further with each breath. ▶ Walk your hands forward until your elbows are straight. Hold for 10 seconds and continue to breathe deeply. To release, slowly uncurl your spine until you are in an upright position. Slowly bring your legs together and relax your spine.

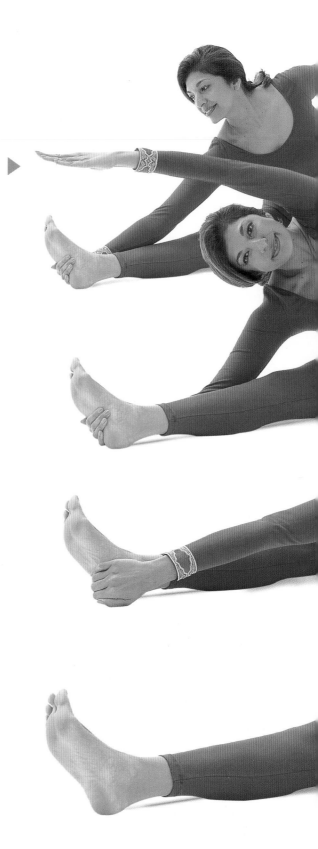

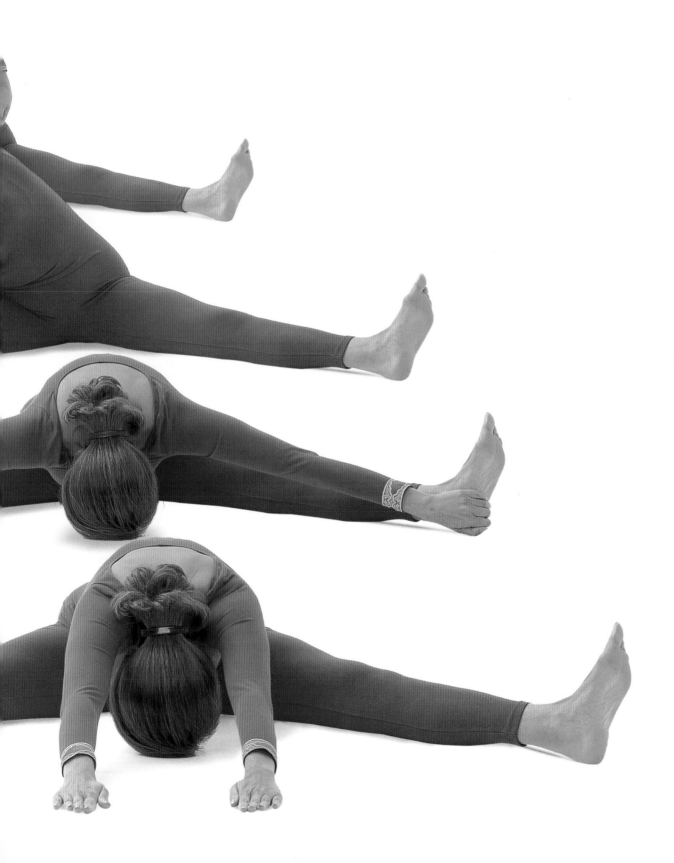

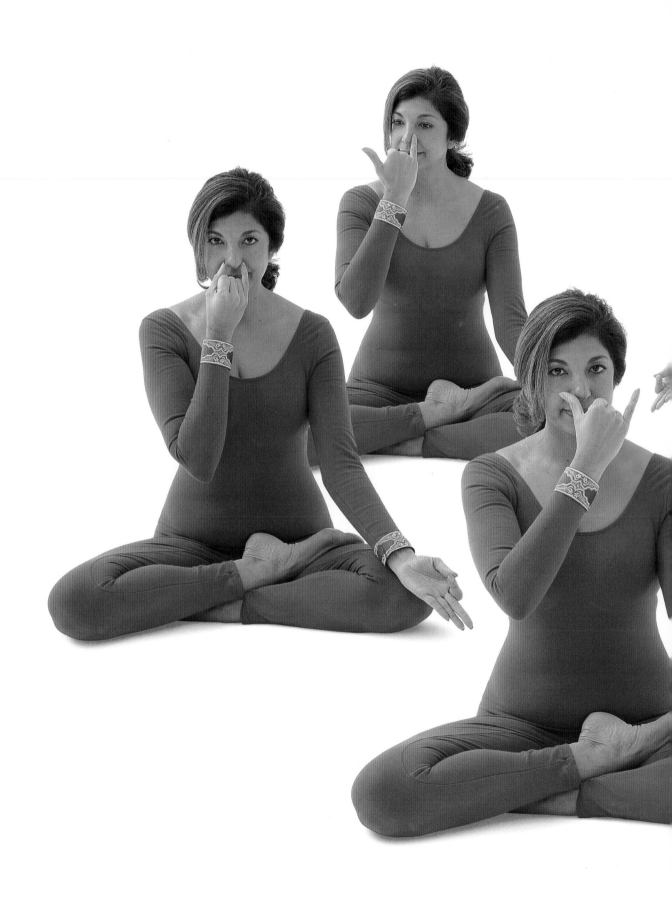

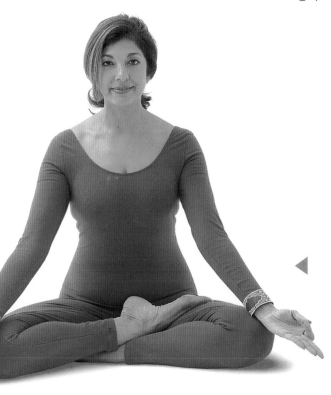

Alternate Nostril Breathing

Pranayama is a Sanskrit word which means 'the science of breath control'. When you learn these breathing techniques you also learn to train and discipline the mind. In yoga you always breathe through your nose from the diaphragm, filling your lungs to capacity, which oxygenates the bloodstream and rejuvenates the cells. This breathing technique balances and harmonizes the masculine and feminine energies in the body. Everyone has both energies and it is important to equalize and unblock the flow of energy, or *prana*.

Begin by sitting tall in a cross-legged, half-lotus, or full lotus position. Open your palms upward and place your hands on your knees. Place your thumb and first finger together. Concentrating on the breath, inhale and exhale deeply, keeping the breath pattern even. Hold this position and breathe for 60 seconds. ▶ Fold your first, second, and third fingers into your right palm and extend your thumb and little finger. Use the little finger to block your left nostril and inhale and exhale only from your right nostril for 10 seconds. ▶ Block your right nostril with your thumb and breathe for 10 seconds through the left nostril only. ▶ Now block the left nostril as before and inhale through the right nostril for 3 seconds. Hold the breath for 3 seconds and then block the right nostril and slowly exhale through the left nostril for 5–6 seconds. Inhale through the left nostril and repeat the exercise at least 10 times.

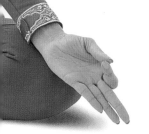

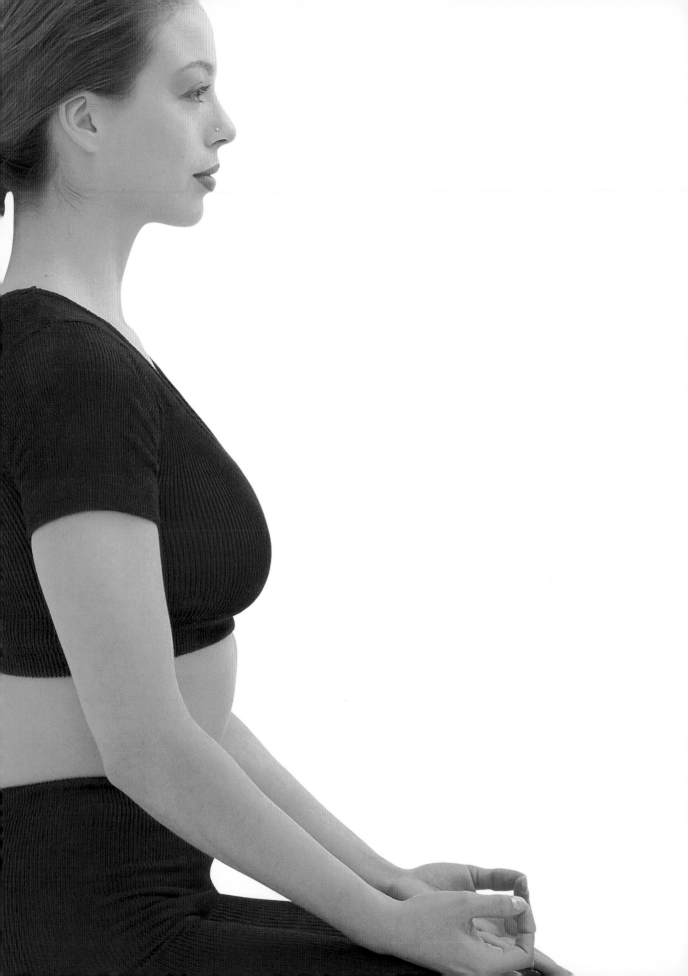

Prelude

There is deep communication between partners who have an understanding of the philosophy of yoga, as yoga-controlled relationships achieve a high quality of cultural and spiritual life. Deep satisfaction steadies and tranquilizes the mind, as well as promoting feelings of love and consideration; Tantric sex will accelerate these emotions and will raise the conscious level of both partners.

The techniques of Tantra were originally used by the sages and mystics to reach Nirvana, or union with God. The aim was to take the basic energy or sex energy from the base chakra and transform it to spiritual energy. Ritualistic practices were learned to raise the conscious level to a higher plane. One of the secrets of Tantra was to know how to arouse different parts of the body and play the partner's body like an instrument to create notes and sensations. So, using the arts of Tantra, two people aimed to work together to raise the sound of their bodies and their vibrations.

Even today, Tantric practices can be used by ordinary people who wish to experience mystical or ecstatic sex. One of the techniques in reaching this goal is total abstinence from sex. The couple sit directly across from one another and keep their eyes fixed on each other. As they breathe deeply their sexual vibrations unite and with meditation they begin to raise together their energy through all chakras to the crown to connect with the cosmic vibration. This gives a feeling of divine bliss and harmony with the universe.

The Tree

The Tree teaches you how to focus and concentrate your mind. Most people think it is very simple to stand on one leg for a length of time without falling over, but it is not as easy as it looks. Many people's minds are very scattered, running through irrelevant thoughts and images, and they are never given a chance to see whether they can give their full attention to one thought or action.

This is an excellent exercise to practise with your partner to help stabilize balance and concentration. Begin by standing in perfect posture as described in the Warm Up (see page 18). ▶ Place your right foot next to your left ankle. Put your palms together to help center your balance. Remember to keep lifting the muscle above the kneecap of your left leg to stop the ankle from moving sideways. ▶ Lift your right foot higher into the inner thigh, resting your left arm on your partner to help you balance. ▶ Lift your arms high above your head, using your partner's support for balance and taking care not to lift your shoulders. Your ultimate goal is to hold for 10 seconds without moving until you can hold the pose by yourself. Repeat on the other leg and let your partner try the whole exercise.

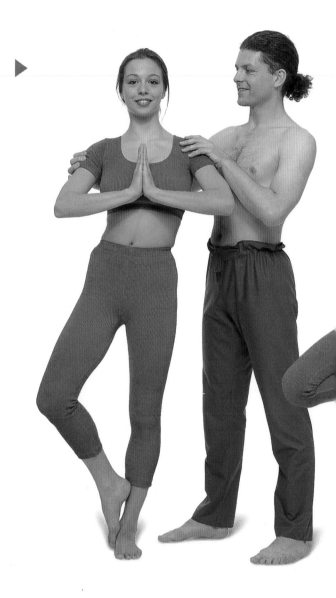

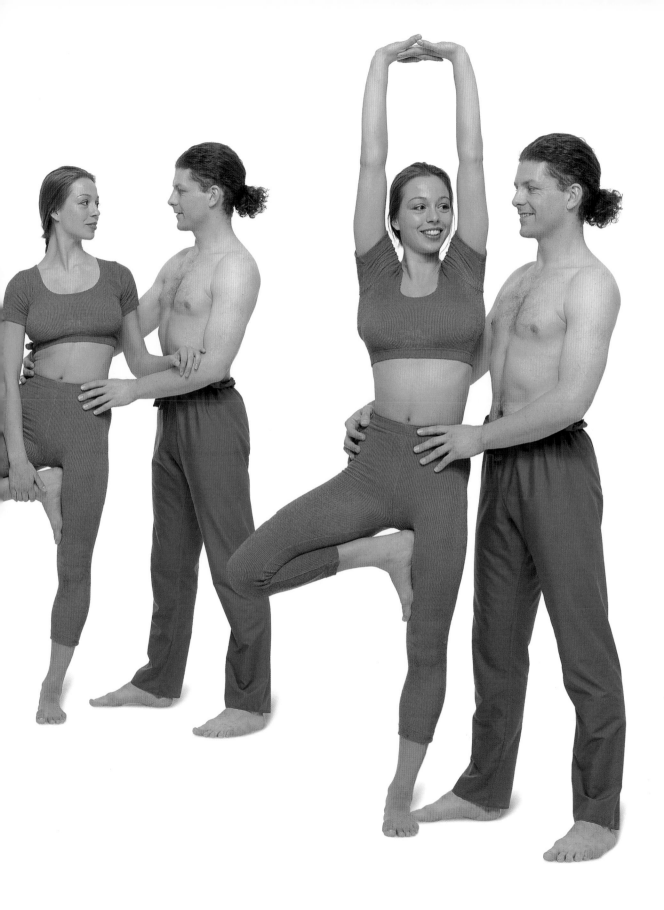

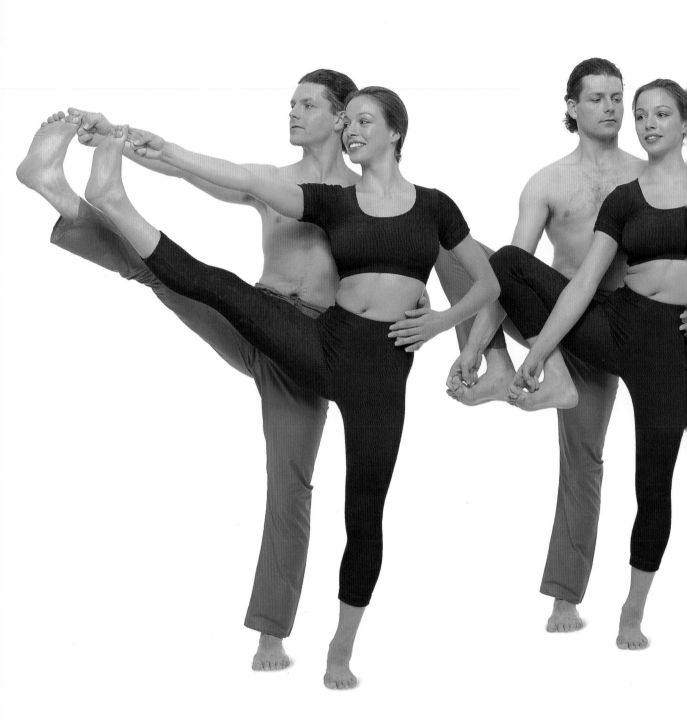

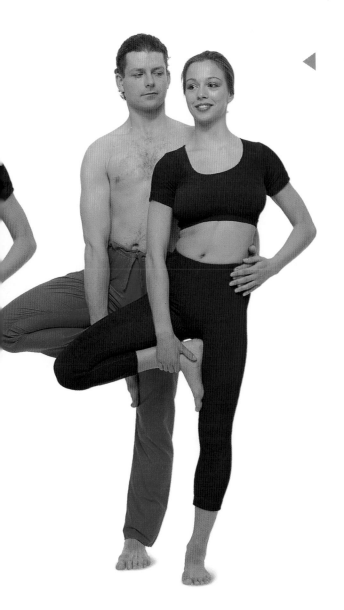

Leg Pull

The Leg Pull is an extension of the Tree. It requires a great deal of practice to perfect as it combines increased flexibility and stamina with concentration. It is a challenging exercise and you should not be surprised if you and your partner fall down; it is always very important when you are practising yoga to maintain your sense of humor! It is an enjoyable and exhilarating feeling to master a particularly difficult exercise and it is great fun to practise with your partner. The Leg Pull also promotes positive thinking and this attitude helps to boost the confidence and self-esteem that are necessary for a good relationship.

Begin the exercise by both partners standing together in perfect posture as described in the Warm Up (see page 18). ▶ Place your left hand on your waist, inhale and lift your right foot up to the inner thigh of your left leg. Exhale and hold for 5 seconds. ▶ Inhale and take your first two fingers around your toe. Exhale and hold the position for 5 seconds, standing as tall as you can. ▶ Inhale and as you exhale extend the leg outward. Keep the hips in line and try not to cave in the chest; the standing leg must remain straight. If you cannot extend the raised leg fully, keep it bent. With increased flexibility and practice you will eventually be able to hold the position for at least 7 full seconds. Release, bend the right leg in a 90-degree angle and return to perfect posture. Repeat on the other side.

The Standing Bow

This exercise is called the Standing Bow because of the beautiful arch that is created by the spine. It is known as the dancer's pose because of the grace and poise that it instills. You feel as if you are about to fly and it is an exhilarating sensation to hold the position while the energy swirls around your body in a circular motion. The Standing Bow steadies your gaze, increases your energy and improves your circulation, while enhancing your sensuality.

Begin the exercise standing with your feet together in perfect posture as described in the Warm Up (see page 18). ▶ Take your left arm upward next to your ear and pull your right leg up behind you, taking hold of the right inner foot. Breathe normally. ▶ Inhale and lift the right leg up behind you, creating an arch in the spine. Keep the left arm straight with the fingertips together in line with your shoulder. ▶ Exhale and continue to stretch further. Breathe deeply as you slowly stretch your body forward, lifting your right leg up as high as possible. Your toes should be over the center of your head to ensure that your hips are square. Try to create a right angle with your arm and standing leg and make sure to keep your chin and head up, with your gaze forward. Hold for as long as you can. Repeat on the other side. Now let your partner try the entire exercise. After you have practised this exercise, ask your partner to stand close by as you attempt to do the exercise on your own.

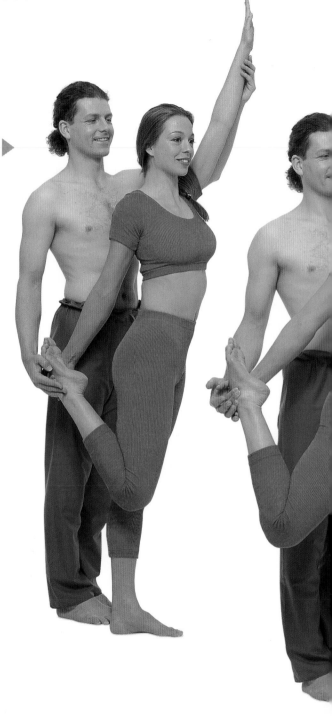

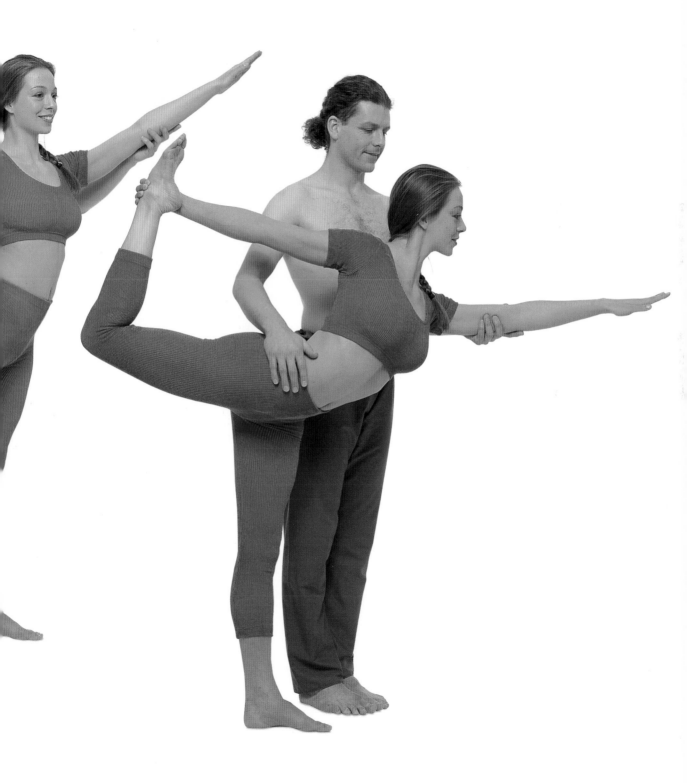

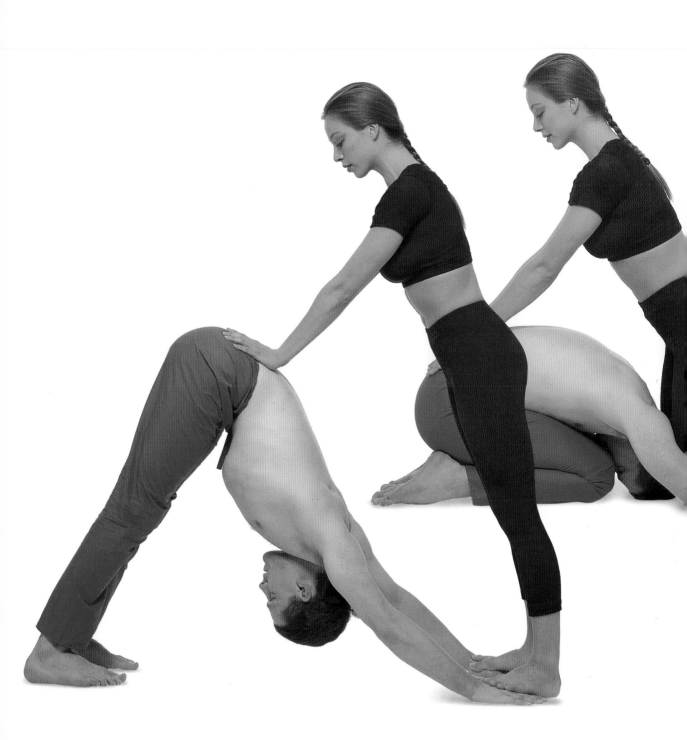

The Dog Pose

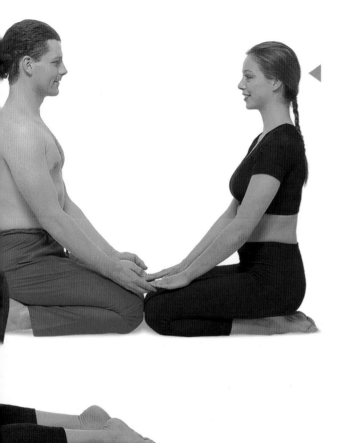

The Dog Pose calms and soothes the nervous system while stretching and toning the entire spine. It is an intense stretch and you can feel every muscle working from your toes and heels through the back of your legs and the base of your spine to the top of your head. As you push the palms of your hands down to the floor you will strengthen your arm muscles and build stamina in the entire body. In the beginning, depending on your fitness level, you may tire easily so it is better to return to position 2 to avoid strain. This is an excellent exercise to assist your partner in achieving a better stretch to increase energy levels and cure fatigue.

Begin by kneeling and facing each other, knees together and feet tucked under. ▶ Breathing normally, relax and drop your forehead down to the floor. Relax your arms down on the floor in front of you on either side of your head. Let your partner kneel by your head, gently pushing the small of your back and hips down to the heels. ▶ Inhale and push up high on to your toes. Exhale and drop your heels as much as possible, ideally to the floor. Straighten your arms and push your palms down to the floor. Breathe deeply as you keep your spine straight and stretch your head down to the floor and toward your knees. To increase your stretch, let your partner stand on your hands and push his or her weight on to your lower back to straighten the spine. Hold for at least 5 seconds. Your goal is to increase the time you hold this pose to 30 seconds or more. Change partners and repeat the entire exercise.

The Warrior

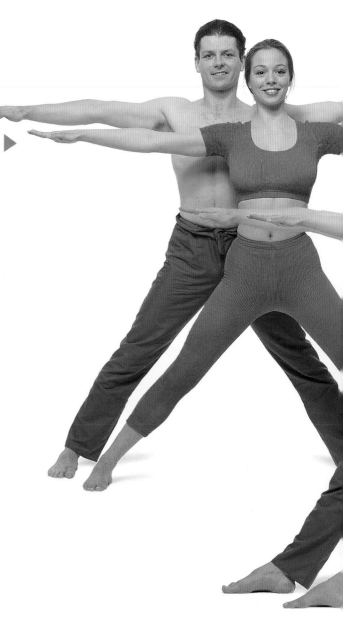

The Warrior is a dynamic pose that creates confidence and powerful energy. There needs to be a vigorous flow of energy between the two partners to balance any negative blockages that may exist – you should feel as if you are one person as you move from one position to another. The deep stretches will release all tension trapped in the body and will build strength and stamina while improving suppleness and flexibility. Some people feel dizzy and nauseous when they begin deep stretching because of the immediate increase of oxygen to the brain as well as the removal of toxins from the kidneys, liver, and spleen. Throughout the series, always breathe deeply and evenly through the nose from the diaphram. The positions look simple but are quite strenuous because of the slow and deliberate pace at which they should be performed. Every time you practise this pose, try to extend the time that you remain in each position to help you build sexual power and dexterity.

Stand tall next to your partner, feet pointed forward and arms outstretched to the sides. Keep your elbows straight and fingertips together. ▶ Breathe normally and turn your right foot to the right in line with the instep of your left foot. ▶ Inhale deeply and as you exhale bend the right knee in a 90-degree angle. Make sure your knee is in a direct line above your heel and does not move forward of your toes as this may cause strain to the knee. Instead widen your stance and take the left leg out further. Continue to breathe deeply and hold for 7 seconds.

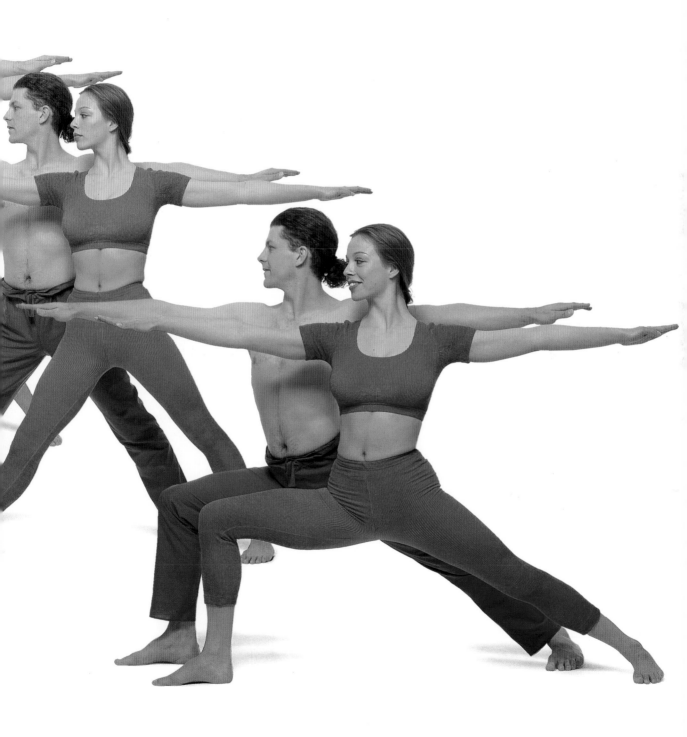

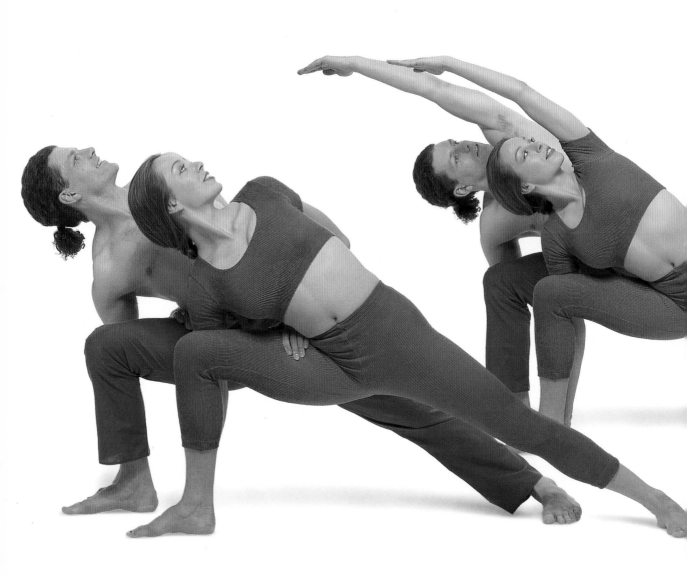

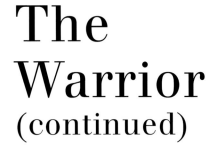

The Warrior (continued)

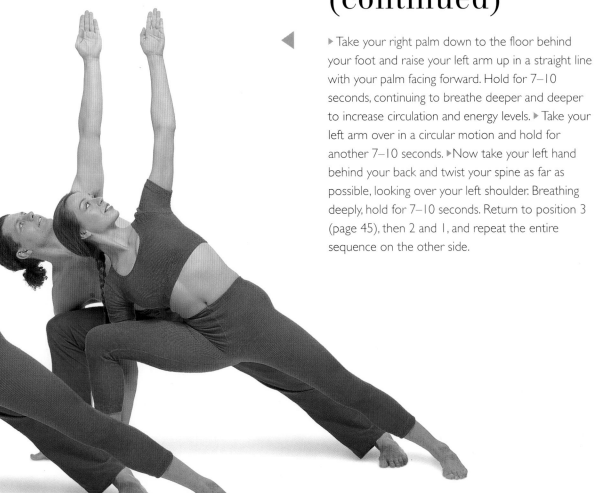

▶ Take your right palm down to the floor behind your foot and raise your left arm up in a straight line with your palm facing forward. Hold for 7–10 seconds, continuing to breathe deeper and deeper to increase circulation and energy levels. ▶ Take your left arm over in a circular motion and hold for another 7–10 seconds. ▶Now take your left hand behind your back and twist your spine as far as possible, looking over your left shoulder. Breathing deeply, hold for 7–10 seconds. Return to position 3 (page 45), then 2 and 1, and repeat the entire sequence on the other side.

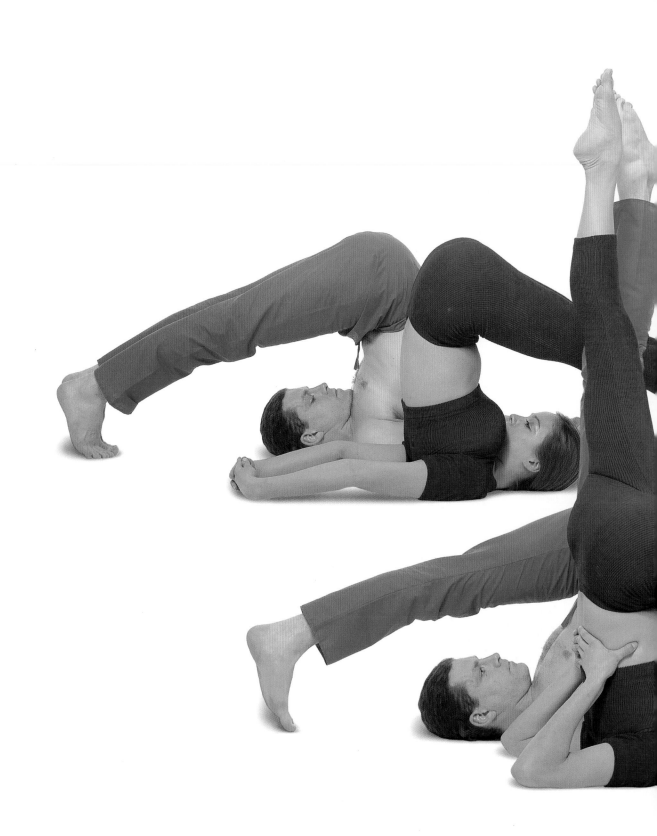

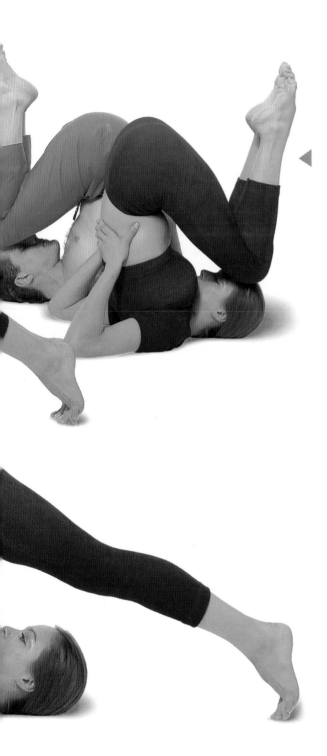

The Plough

This exercise increases the flexibility of the spine and strengthens and tones the back. It is an inverted position that allows the blood to flow down to the internal organs, which replenishes and recharges all the cells. It helps to calm and soothe the nervous system as well as releasing tension in the neck and shoulders. When the chin is locked into the chest it stimulates and regulates the thyroid gland, which stabilizes the metabolism and hormonal levels of the body. This will keep your weight constant and your temperament free of mood swings. Do not practise the Plough if you are pregnant or have a heavy menstrual flow.

Begin the Plough by lying flat on your back with your arms at your sides. Breathe normally. Inhale and lift your knees into your chest. Exhale and as you inhale roll back your knees toward your head, bringing your hands to your waist to support your lower back, and place your knees to your forehead. Exhale and breathe normally. Make sure to point your toes. ▸Now straighten your legs and stretch them out behind your head as far as possible. Tuck your toes under and keep your breath even and deep. ▸ Inhale and lift your right leg up in a straight line to your partner. Point your toes and hold together for 5–15 seconds. Change legs and repeat. To finish, return to position 2, then 1 and gently roll down until you are lying flat down on the floor again. Breathe deeply and relax for 60 seconds.

Head to the Knee

This pose lengthens and tones the entire spine and relaxes the brain. It opens the hips and strengthens the leg muscles. All forward bends help to release toxins that are trapped in the system and this forward action stimulates the kidneys, liver, and pancreas. When you first begin this exercise you might feel disappointed that you are unable to bend very far, but with continued practice and correct breathing you will be surprised at how flexible your spine becomes. Never push or jerk your body to increase the stretch as this might cause strain to your muscles; as you increase the depth of your breathing you will automatically relax and this will loosen tight muscles in the legs and lower back and you will stretch even further. Keep your feet firmly placed on the floor and distribute your weight evenly between your heels and toes. As you stretch forward, think of moving your spine out from your tailbone. This will help to flatten and lengthen the spine.

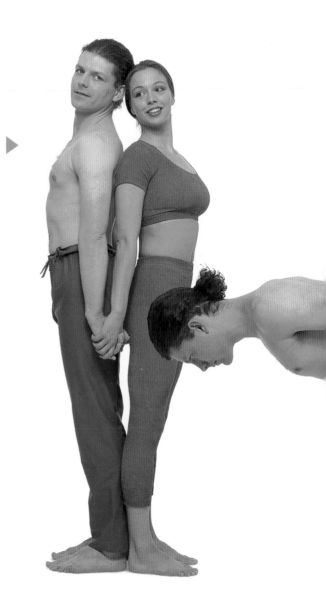

Stand tall back-to-back with your partner and check to make sure you are in perfect posture (see page 18). Breathe normally and hold hands to give each other support. ▶ Inhale, keeping your spine as flat as possible, then exhale and bend forward halfway. Hold for 5 seconds while you breathe normally. ▶Take a deep breath and as you exhale drop your head down to your knees. Continue to breathe deeply and hold this position for 30 seconds. To release, inhale slowly, bend the knees, curl the spine and gently unroll it until you have reached the first position. Repeat the entire exercise once.

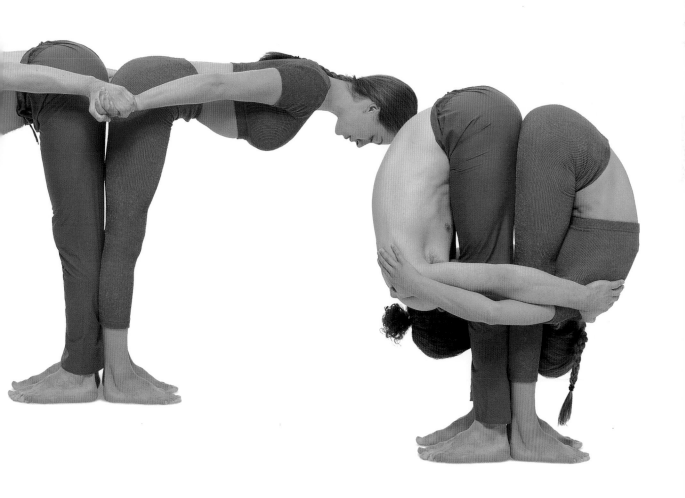

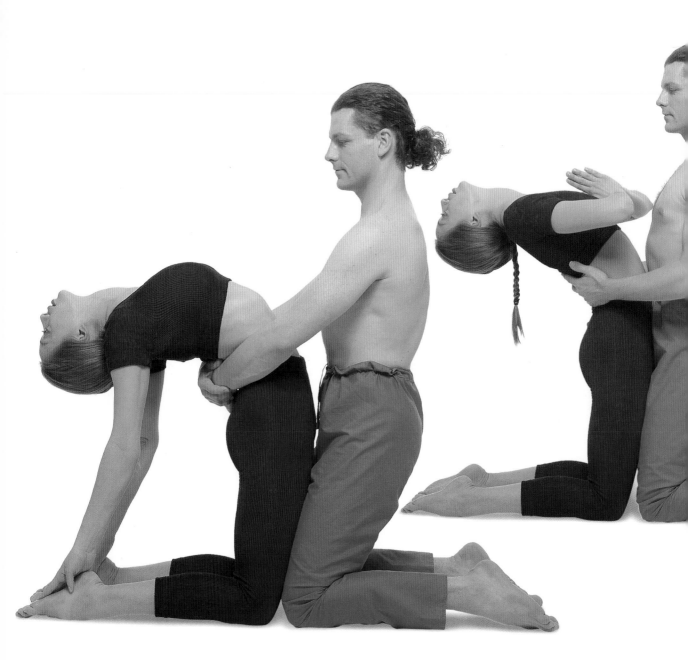

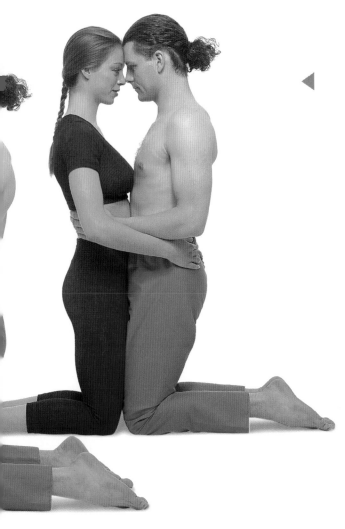

The Camel

This is an intense back bend that tones the entire spine and every muscle in the body. The flexibility required in lovemaking is greatly improved and the increased circulation helps vitality and prevents the signs of ageing. Many people dislike the idea of bending backward, but it is very liberating to toss your head back, open your chest and throat and push your hips forward. The Camel becomes less daunting to learn when you have your partner's help because as you share the experience you will build mutual respect and trust for each other.

Begin by kneeling in front of your partner. Let your partner secure both arms around your waist so you feel confident of his or her support. ▶Inhale deeply and as you exhale push your hips forward as much as possible, shifting your weight into your hips; make sure you do not cheat and distribute your weight into your legs and thighs. Your hips should be in a direct line to your knees. Slowly drop your head back and arch your back as much as possible. Place your hands together in a prayer pose and open your throat. Make sure your face is relaxed, especially in the jaw and around the eyes. ▶ Your partner should now hold your lower back even more strongly while you take your hands down to your heels. Keep pushing your hips forward to increase the stretch in the back. Say 'Aaah' in a deep, constant tone – if you are unable to do so it means that you are still tense. Breathe deeply and relax in this pose for a minimum of 10 seconds. To release, sit back onto the floor between your feet and relax your forehead down to the floor. Breathe deeply and relax for 15 seconds. This position will counteract the back bend to ensure there is no strain in the back. Change with your partner and repeat the entire exercise.

The Locust

A good sexual performance demands a very strong back, especially in the ardent poses of the *Kama Sutra*. The Locust not only helps to alleviate back pain but strengthens the back and legs so you are able to build endurance and stamina. It also helps improve your posture by strengthening the lower back so you are able to sit and stand for a length of time. It is important to learn to isolate certain muscle groups and in this exercise, even though every muscle is working, there is an emphasis on the stomach, legs, and buttocks. Do not worry if you cannot lift your legs very high behind you because it is more important that your shoulder blades and hipbones remain on the floor to ensure that your spine is in correct alignment. As you practise this pose you will be able to lift your leg higher. Think of stretching your leg out from the hipbone and make sure you do not rock from side to side.

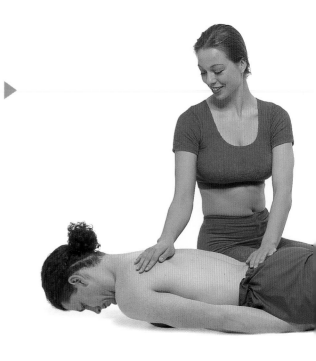

Begin the exercise by lying face down on the floor, your hands under your hipbones. Your partner should watch to see that your spine is perfectly straight. ▶Inhale, and raise your right leg off the floor. Exhale, breathe normally and hold for 5 seconds. Exhale and slowly lower the leg down to the floor. Inhale, raise the left leg and hold for 5 seconds. Exhale and slowly lower the left leg. Repeat. ▶Ask your partner to make sure both hips are down to the floor, then take a deep inhalation and raise both legs. Hold for 5–10 seconds. Exhale and slowly lower both legs. This is quite a strenuous exercise and your heartbeat should be racing. Relax and turn your head to one side until your pulse is normal. Repeat the entire exercise.

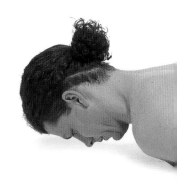

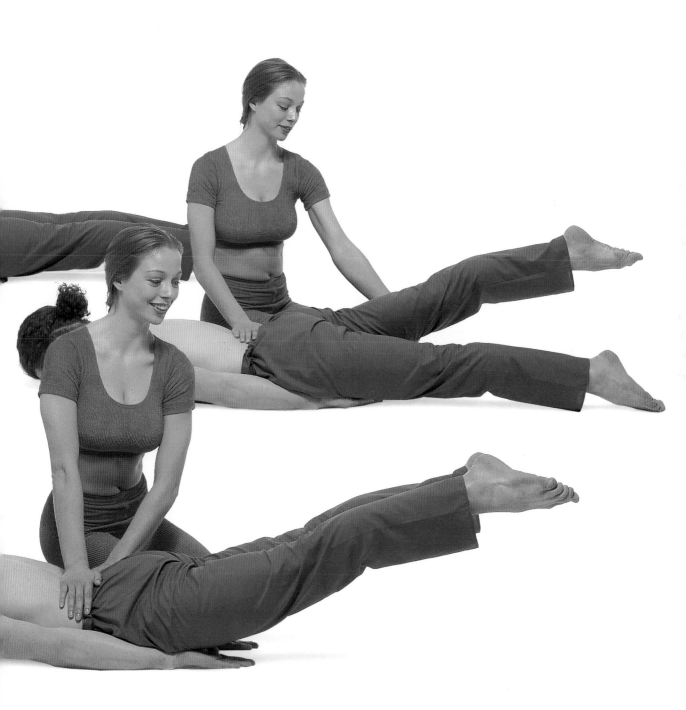

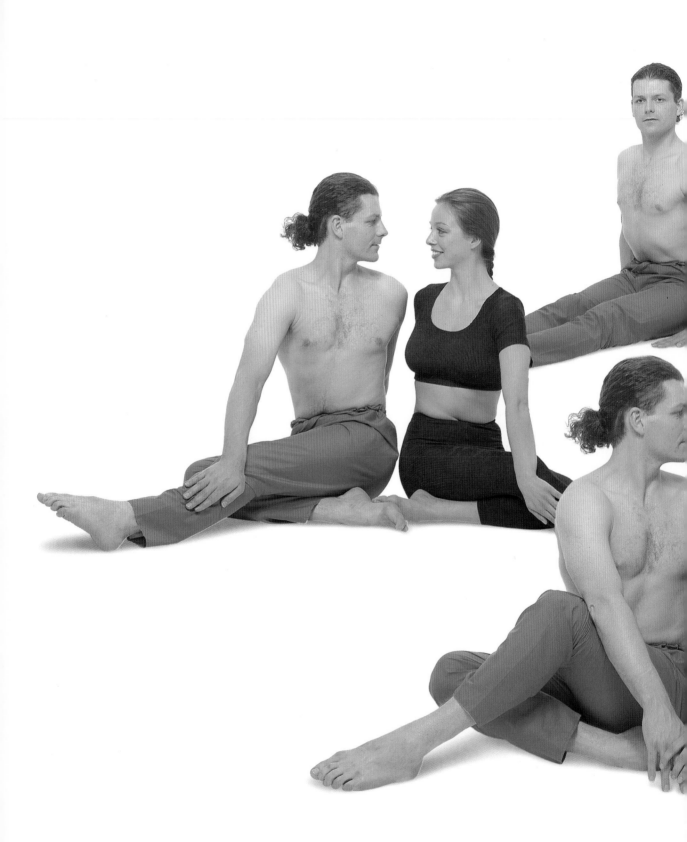

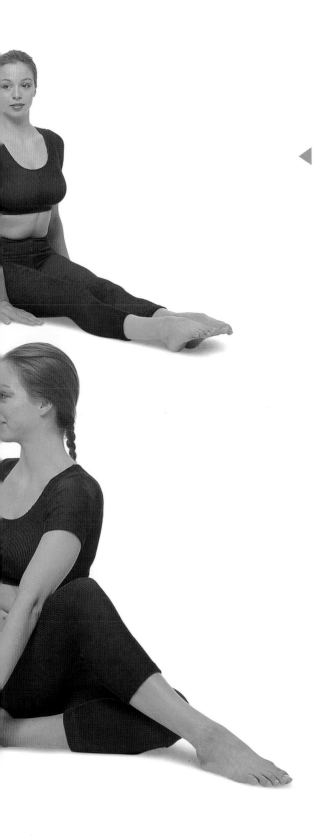

Sitting Twist

All twists are excellent for increasing flexibility of the spine and eliminating toxins from the system. They are very effective in relieving backaches and headaches as well as stiffness in the neck and shoulders. As the upper body turns, the kidneys and abdominal organs are activated, aiding digestion and removing sluggishness. The beauty of twists is that there is no final position because as you become more supple your twist increases. There are many variations to the classic twist, but all alleviate back pain and inflexibility of the lower back. It is a great pleasure to hear the clicks in the spine when you release tension. You cannot be a good sex partner if you are full of anxieties and this twist eliminates the stresses and strains that build up in the body. The most important thing is to know for sure that you wish to rid yourself of tension. Once you have won the first battle with your mind, your body will follow. Think of the joy it will bring you when you release your mind and body from trapped energy.

Sit up as tall as possible with your legs extended in front of you, side-to-side but facing slightly away from each other. ▶ Both of you then bend the outer leg to create a 90-degree angle with your knee and hip. ▶ Take the outer arm across in front of the inner knee and gently twist the spine. ▶ Lift the inner leg up and place the foot in front of the outer knee. Continue to stretch as far as possible. Breathe as deeply as you can and relax into the stretch. Hold for up to 60 seconds. Change sides and repeat.

Leg Stretch

In lovemaking it is so important to trust your partner even if the poses are difficult. There is a healthy give and take in this pose which will give you both a sense of balancing and harmonizing each other's energy in preparation for the sexual poses that follow. This stretch increases the flexibility and suppleness of the spine and strengthens the legs and back. It also stretches and tones the internal organs. Because you are putting your full weight onto each other you are helping your partner stretch forward without strain while you are working on stretching your entire body backward and opening the chest. In yoga, the importance of opening the chest is to steady the emotional center or heart chakra that lies just below the physical heart. The final position opens this center and stabilizes emotional disturbances. The mind becomes still as if you were in a meditative pose.

Sit tall back-to-back with your legs outstretched, pointing your toes in front of you. ▶ Bring your knees up while keeping your feet flat on the floor. Lean back onto your partner's upper back so he or she will automatically move forward. Push down your feet to the floor, raise your hips and lean back even further. ▶ Stretch your legs out fully and place your entire weight onto your partner's spine, arching your back. Take your arms over your head to increase the stretch. This movement will help your partner stretch forward, placing the forehead down to the knees. If the flexibility of the partners is unequal you can modify the pose by not putting your total weight onto the other person. Change positions with your partner and repeat the entire exercise.

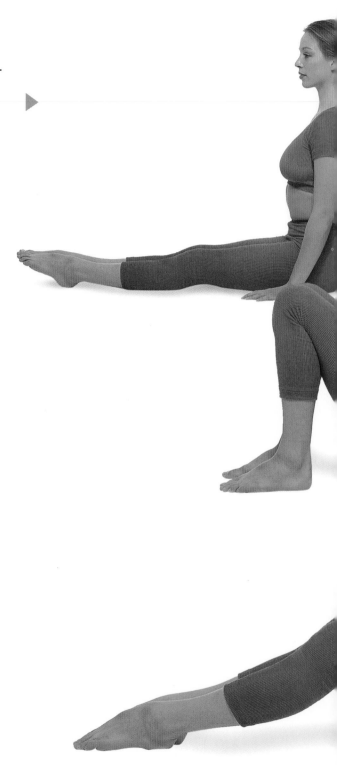

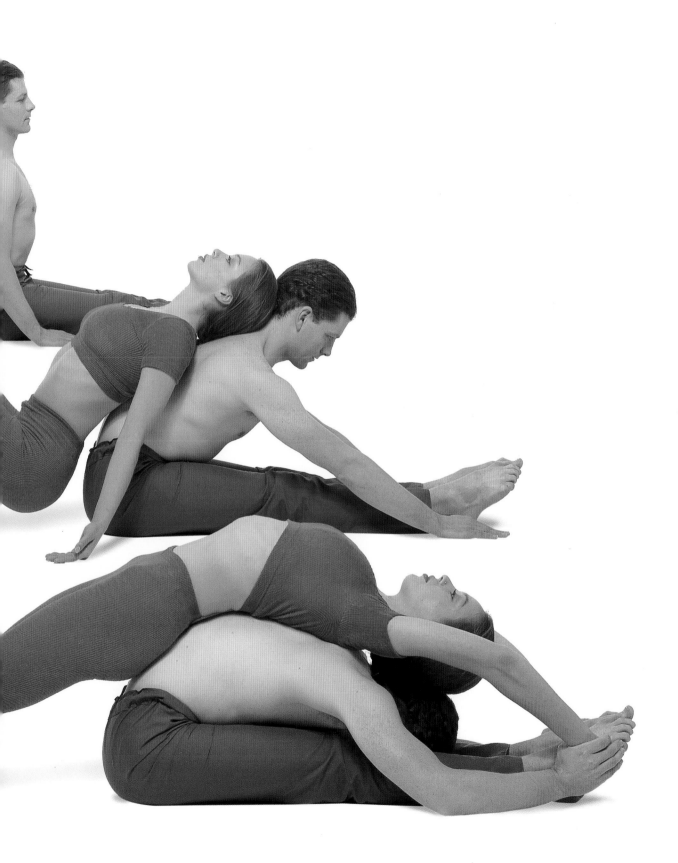

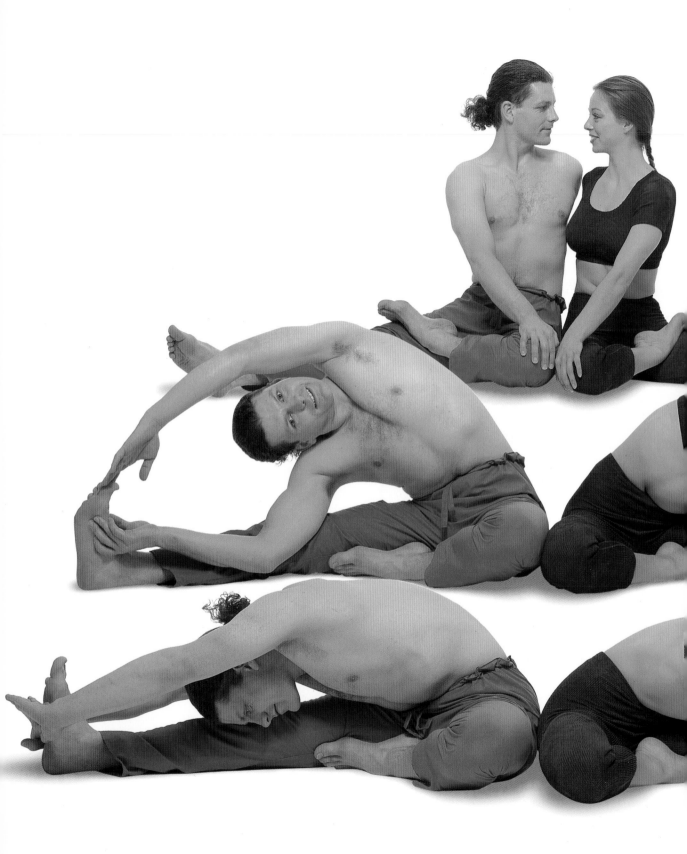

Half Lotus Side Stretch

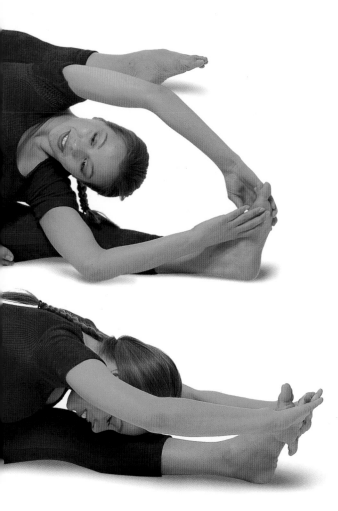

This pose is an excellent exercise for toning your entire body and calming your central nervous system. In yoga exercises you are continually moving your whole body in every direction: forward, backward, sideways. This twisting and turning of the spine strengthens the nerves and helps build the immune system. A healthy sex life is based on good health generally and when you feel well you will perform better. As you stretch to the side and front in this exercise, try not to collapse your spine. Always stretch from the tailbone and elongate each muscle to eliminate the fat around each muscle group. The result will be a lean, muscular body that is tight and firm.

Begin these stretches by sitting back-to-back as you did in the Leg Stretch (see page 58). Breathe normally. Place your right foot on the left thigh or left foot on the right thigh in the Half Lotus and twist your spine to look at your partner. Slide your bent leg down to the floor, keeping your knee in line with your hip. ▶ Inhale and stretch over the outstretched leg. Take your upper arm over your head close to your ear and lower your other arm to the floor. Exhale and take your fingertips to clasp your feet. Breathe normally and hold the position for 10 seconds. ▶ Now face your extended knee. Inhale, and stretch forward so your forehead touches your knee. Exhale and clasp your hands together behind your feet. Breathe deeply and evenly and hold this position for 10 seconds or for as long as you feel comfortable. Change sides and repeat the entire sequence.

Back Arch

This Back Arch immediately restores vitality and energy to the system and relaxes the brain. It also allows you and your partner to help each other improve your suppleness. When your back is arched and your head dropped to the floor behind you the blood rushes to your brain, revitalizing and replenishing your brain cells. It is impossible to be a good lover when your sex drive is low or there is a lack of enthusiasm, and this exercise is an excellent tonic to refresh your mind when you are feeling lethargic and tired. It also allows you to move intimately with your partner which will set the mood for lovemaking. When you are helping each other to stretch, be aware of each other's capabilities – in many cases the flexibility of the couple may not be equal. Never force or push your partner; remember that yoga is non-competitive and everyone should always work at their own pace. With continued practice and patience you will see how fast you progress.

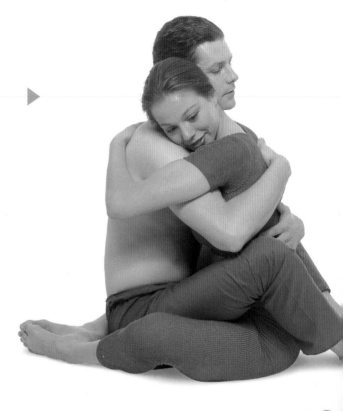

Begin by sitting facing each other and hold one another in a gentle, loving manner. Take your legs over each other's thighs and bring both feet together. ▶ With your partner holding your lower back for support, inhale, arch your back and lift up as high as possible to rest on the top of your head. Exhale and breathe normally. This improves circulation to the face and neck and you will feel the blood flow into the brain. Hold for 5–10 seconds. ▶ Inhale, release the neck and have your partner help you back up. Exhale and relax your spine forward as your partner arches the spine and relaxes backward. Repeat the exercise five times with a back-and-forth motion.

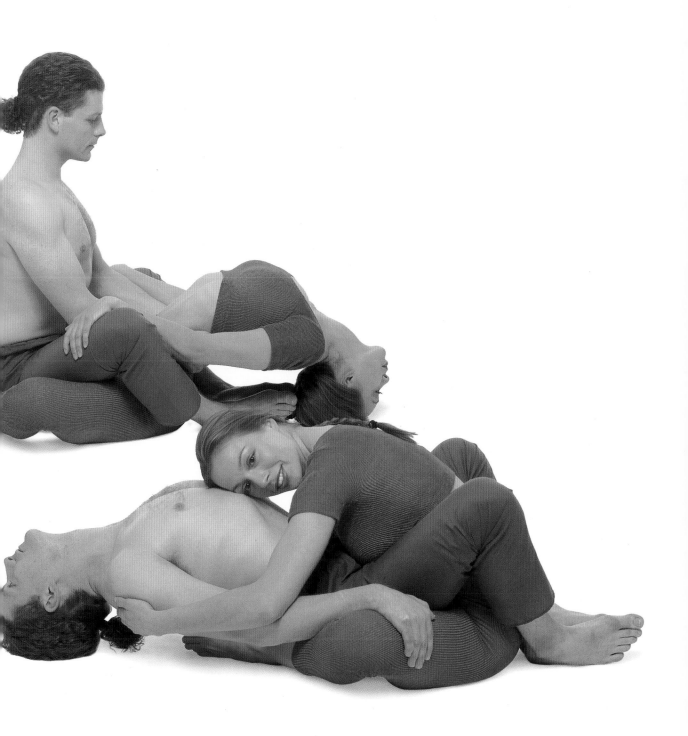

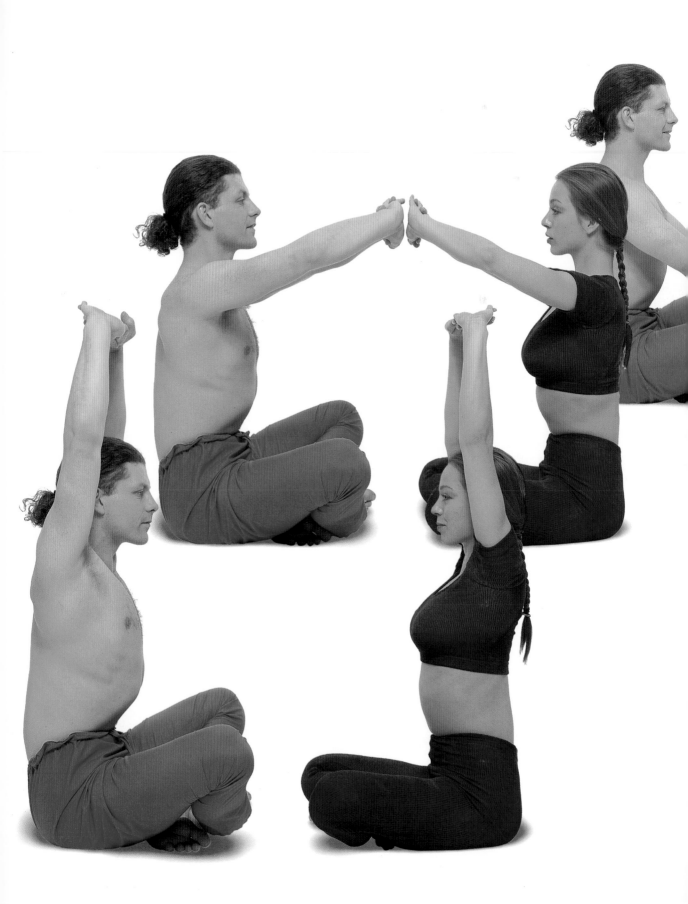

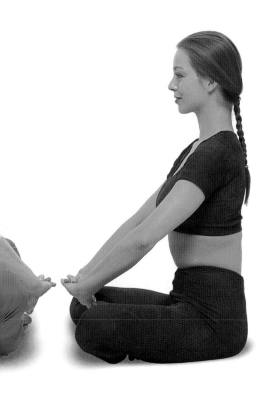

Heart Chakra

It is very important in lovemaking to be in tune mentally and emotionally with your partner. Tantric sex unites your energy centers and it is vital that these centers remain unblocked. There are seven chakras in the body and the heart chakra lies between the breastbone. It is the energy that rules compassion and unconditional love and when this energy is blocked it leads to psychological and emotional disturbances. This exercise balances all seven centers from the base or pelvic region, through the navel into the solar plexus, through the heart into the throat, and through the third eye (between the eyebrows) into the top of the head or crown to unite with the cosmic or universal energy. This technique is used as a ritual in Tantra to arouse sexual passion and heighten sexual pleasure.

Begin by sitting cross-legged, facing each other, with enough distance between you to prevent you from touching each other. ▶ Sit up as tall as possible and clasp your hands together, palms facing outwards. ▶ Concentrating on your base chakra, inhale deeply and slowly raise your arms, moving through each chakra until you raise your arms high over your head. Keep the breath even and continuous as you slowly fill your lungs with air. Exhale and slowly bring the arms back down to position 1. Try to match the exact pace of your partner while performing the exercise. Repeat up to 10 times.

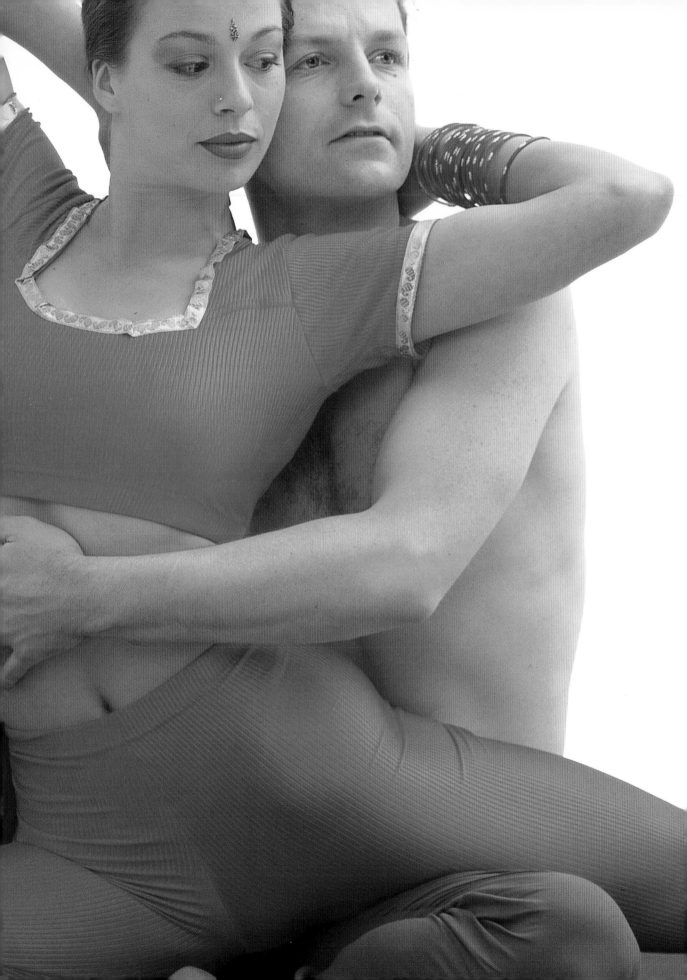

Love Poses

Sexual positions, or Kama asanas, bring variety and
excitement to the sex act. In the *Kama Sutra*, the
great sage Vatsyayana describes the ways to achieve
pleasure through a systematic and scientific
approach to the anatomy of the body and the
reactions of the mind. While the sex urge is a natural
and powerful phenomenon, it can be disciplined by
the gift of yoga.

Within these sexual poses it is important to
prolong the sex act and to increase pleasure by
observing and understanding it. If you are already
acquainted with the yoga positions you will not find
any *Kama Sutra* pose difficult to achieve – in fact, a
path illuminated by the light of yoga will remain
pure and bright, even when it leads to the fulfilment
of Kama or sexual bliss. To condemn knowledge of
sex as a sin, and to glorify ignorance as bliss, merely
promotes misery, incompetence, fear, and damage
to the psyche. No man should think of sexual
intercourse as the supreme test of his manliness, nor
should a woman regard it as her badge of femininity.
If you feel an act of sex to be a test or competition
the spontaneity and the naturalness of the situation
will be destroyed. Embrace it as a wonderful and
integral part of a healthy and rounded life and enjoy
the pleasure that is a fundamental right for each
human being.

The
Warrior

'The dynamic warrior beholds his beautiful
maiden and wishes to enchant her with
physical pleasure. This noble man is gentle
but strong and she graceful and poised. As
he swirls her into a passionate embrace
she succumbs to his physical strength and
together they reach divine bliss to unite
with the cosmic universe.'

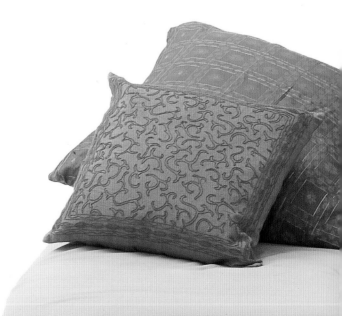

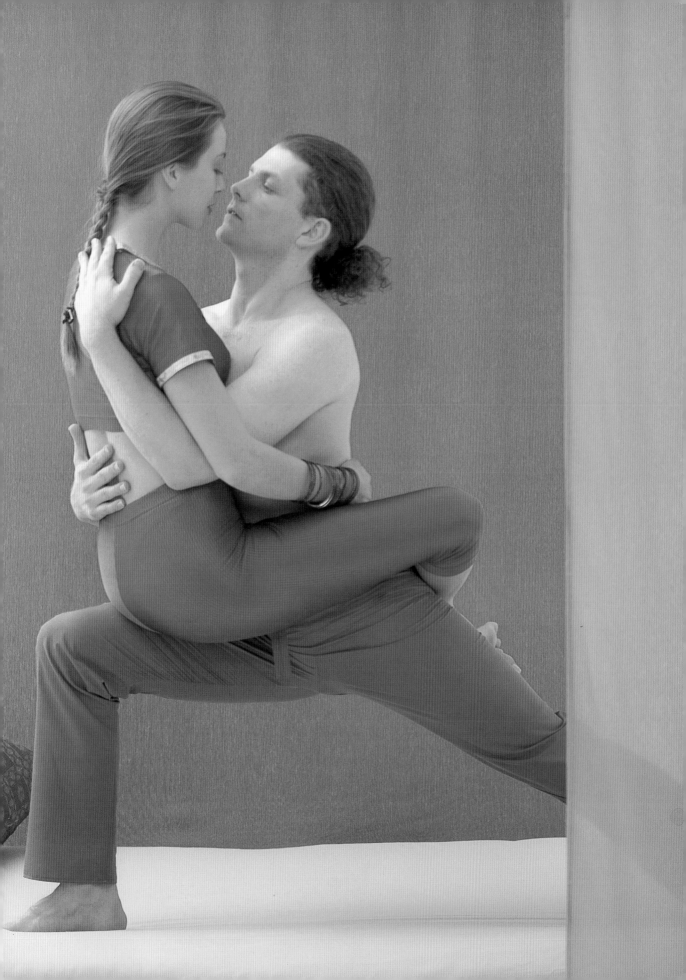

The Warrior Love Pose

Stamina and strength are required by the man for him to be able to hold this position for a length of time. The Balance (see page 22) and the Warrior (see page 44) are both good exercises for building up all the muscles in his legs, especially the ankles, knees, and thighs.

The man begins this pose by standing tall in a wide second position, feet 1–1.2m (3–4ft) apart. Both arms are at his side and his toes are pointed forward. He turns his left foot to the left so his left heel is in a direct line to his right foot. He bends his left knee and lunges, making sure that his knee does not reach forward of his foot – he should create an exact 90-degree angle to the floor. His right leg is extended fully. It is important that both feet are firmly on the ground and his weight is evenly distributed in order to be well balanced. The woman stands close to him. When he is in the Warrior position and is confident of his balance, she places her right foot on his upper thigh. She places her right hand on her waist and puts her left arm around his neck in a loving manner. ▶ Now she swings her body around and sits on his left thigh with her left leg supporting her weight. She clasps both arms around his neck and lifts her right leg around his waist. ▶ When both partners have an equal balance she lifts her left leg up to balance on him completely. It is very important that the woman be poised and graceful. She should feel as light as a feather and the man should feel strong, powerful, and dynamic.

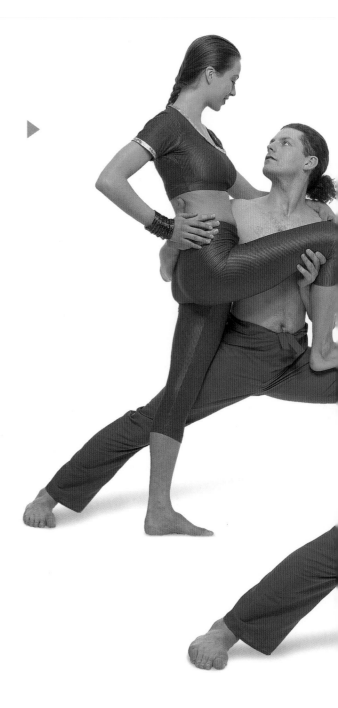

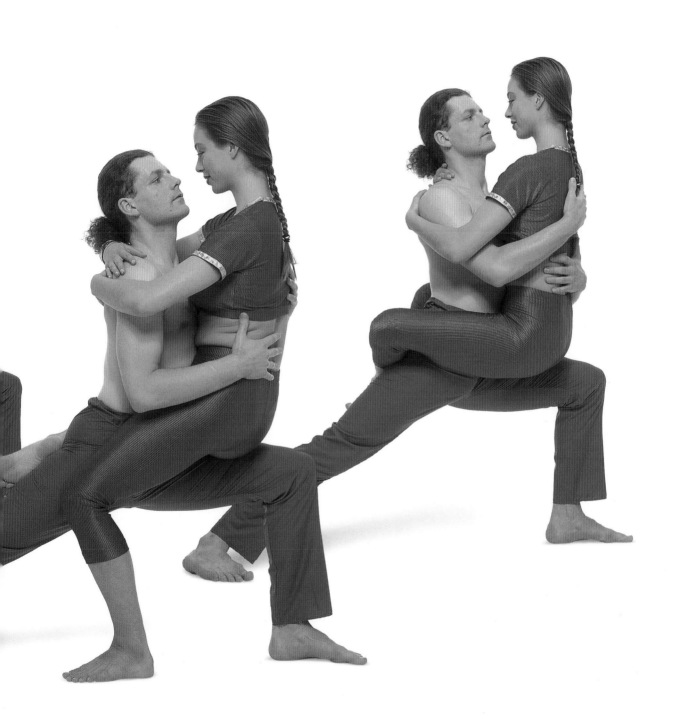

The Tree

'When the roots of love are strong the branches can weather even the most violent storm. In the midst of chaos and destruction the stillness of pleasure is an erotic art that bonds and unites two truly loving souls.'

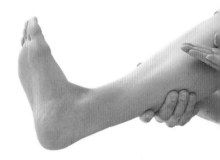

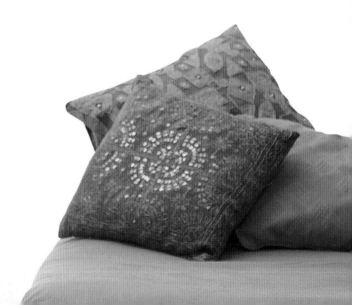

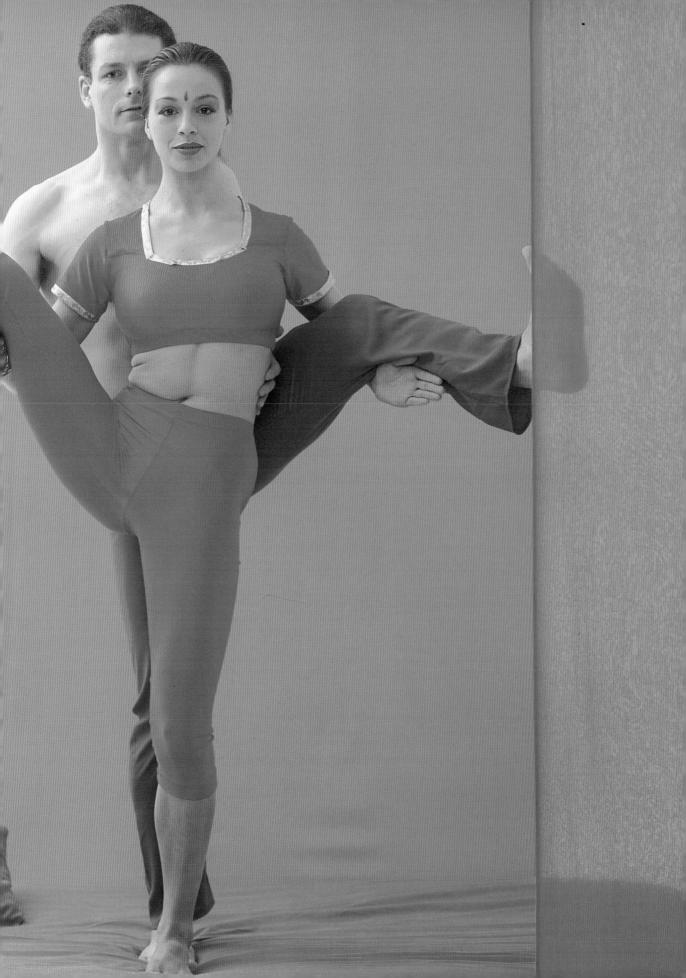

The Tree Love Pose

The couple need to focus their minds in order to execute this difficult love pose. When they practise the Balance (see page 22), the Tree (see page 36) and the Leg Pull (see page 38) they will learn the art of balancing on one leg as well as improving the flexibility of their hips and hamstrings. It is important in this pose to keep the hips square and the standing leg straight to help maintain poise and balance.

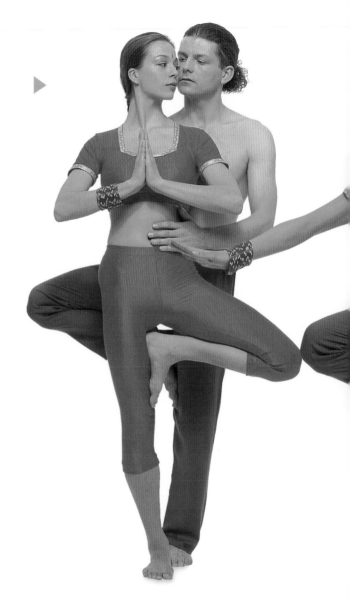

The couple stand together with the woman in front of the man, distributing their weight evenly on each foot. The woman lifts her left leg and places her left foot on her inner right thigh, lifting the muscle above the right knee to stop her ankle shifting sideways. She places her palms together to help steady her balance. The right side of every person, male or female, represents the masculine energy in the body and the left side the feminine; placing the palms together unites and harmonizes these two energies. The man follows his partner on the opposite leg and places his right foot on his left inner thigh. He places his left hand on her midriff to steady her balance and his right arm at his side. As they are not directly looking at one another they steady their gaze on one spot to unite their energies. ▶ The woman now takes her left hand under her thigh behind her knee and lifts her leg up as high as possible while keeping her spine straight. Her right arm extends to balance her weight. The man holds onto her lifted leg. ▶ The man lifts his right leg with his right hand in a direct line to his partner. Both partners can now bend the standing leg slightly. If it is difficult to maintain balance during coitus the man can lean on a wall for support.

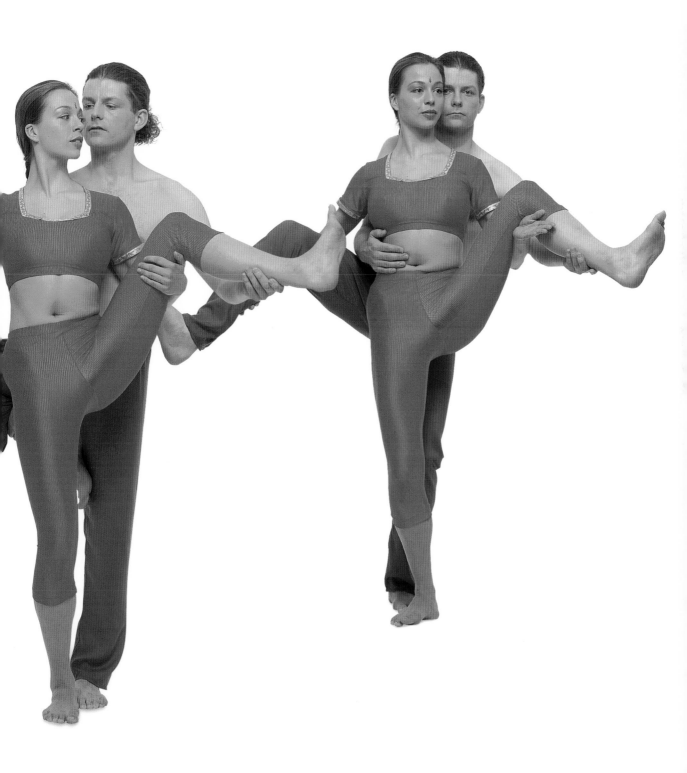

Carry

'To love others is an art and we must know its theory and practices, its methods and techniques, in order to master the art of giving love. If we learn how to love we will certainly be loved by others. Love is an ability, a capacity in our minds, which is to be systematically cultivated. Once the faculty of love has been developed we have a total freedom to love and any situation is a fertile field in which to cultivate this love.'

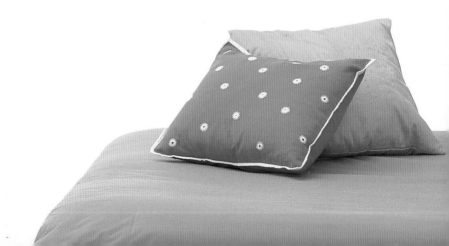

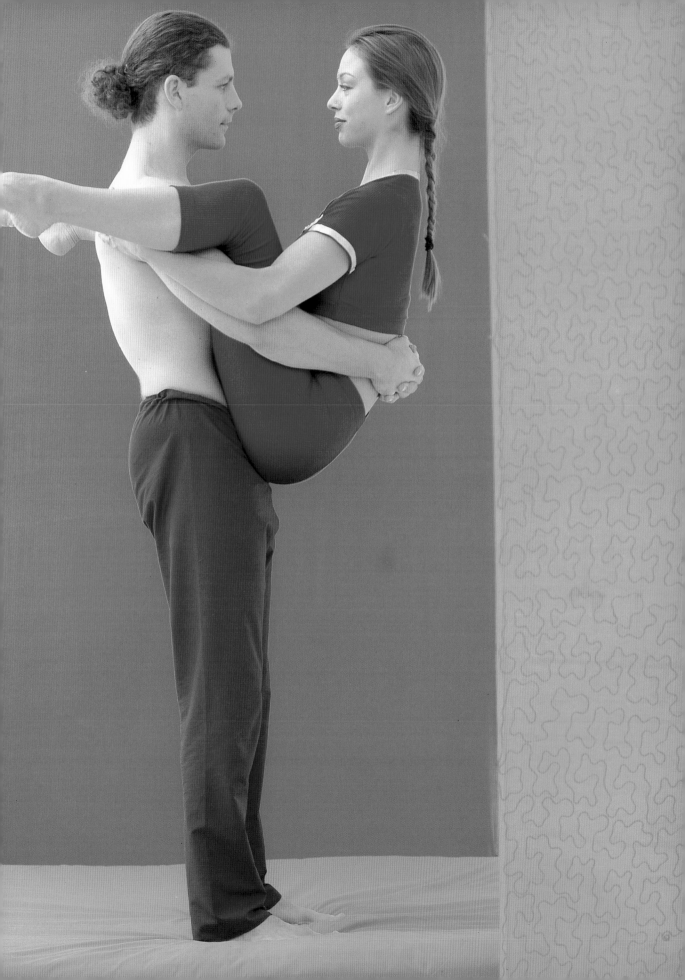

Carry Love Pose

This pose relies on the physical strength of the man and the ability of the woman to trust her partner completely. It is a difficult pose to perform for the first time but with continued practice it can be achieved. In preparation you can build your body strength by learning the Dog Pose (see page 42) and Head to the Knee (see page 50). It is important for the woman to be lithe, and timing the jump will help the man lift her smoothly and effectively. The man needs a strong back and it is important that he bends his knees when he lifts the woman to protect his back from any injury.

The couple stand facing each other with both feet together. The man kneels down in front of the woman and holds on to her waist. She raises her right leg over his left shoulder and puts her left hand around his neck and her right hand on his forearm. ▶ As the man lifts her up she rises high onto her toes and balances on her left foot, looking directly into his eyes. He puts his arms around her, holding the middle of her back to support her, and she gently holds on to his shoulders. ▶ As the man lifts her, the woman simultaneously takes a quick jump and places her left leg over his right shoulder. The man can then easily lift her up and remain in a standing position. The woman slides down his body so her legs are above his elbows and holds onto his arms. He supports her back with both hands on her waist.

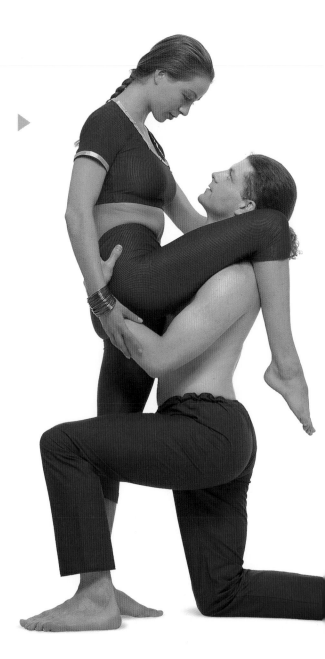

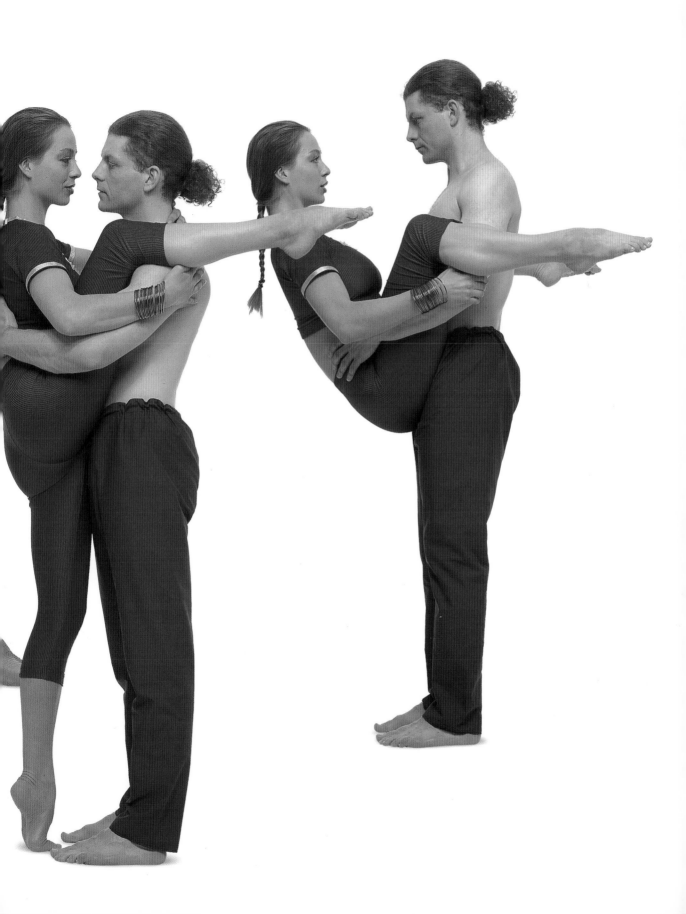

The Wheel

'The quest for love is universal. Man, irrespective of race, creed, language and nationality, seeks and thrives on love but rarely ever finds deep, lasting love. We selfishly only want to receive love and are unwilling to give unconditional love – the only true source of happiness.'

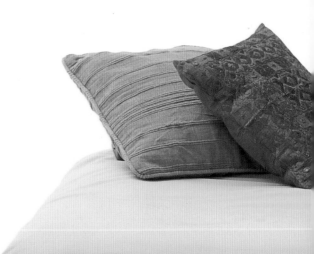

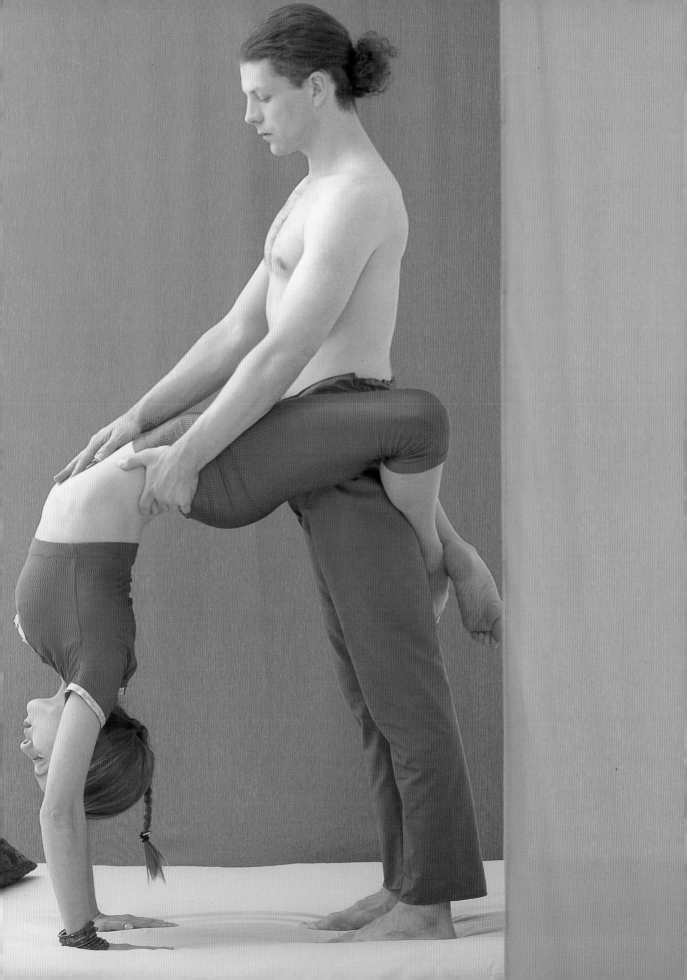

The Wheel Love Pose

This is a dynamic, erotic love pose that requires physical strength, flexibility of the spine, and stamina. It is a great challenge and needs practice and patience to achieve. The Cobra and Bow (see page 28), the Camel (see page 52), the Leg Stretch (see page 58) and the Back Arch (see page 62) are good postures to help build the flexibility and strength of the spine. They will also help to overcome any fear on the woman's part so she can move backward into the pose with confidence.

The woman begins by lying flat on the floor with her feet in line with her hips. She takes her arms over her head so her hands are placed close to her ears on either side of her head. Her fingertips are together and pointing toward her feet. ▶ She inhales and lifts her hips as high as possible off the floor to create a beautiful arch in her spine. She drops her head down in line with her arms. When she is in the correct Wheel position the man kneels down to the floor on his left knee, keeping his right foot in a right angle to the floor. He holds on to his partner's waist to help support her lower back. ▶ He gradually gains her total confidence and then lift her hips off the floor while he bends his knees to protect his back from any strain as he is lifting her. She wraps her right leg around his waist while balancing with her left foot to the floor. ▶ When he has secured her total weight, the woman wraps both legs around the man's waist and crosses her ankles to grip his back. The man straightens his knees and lifts his spine to stand in perfect posture as described in the Warm Up (see page 18).

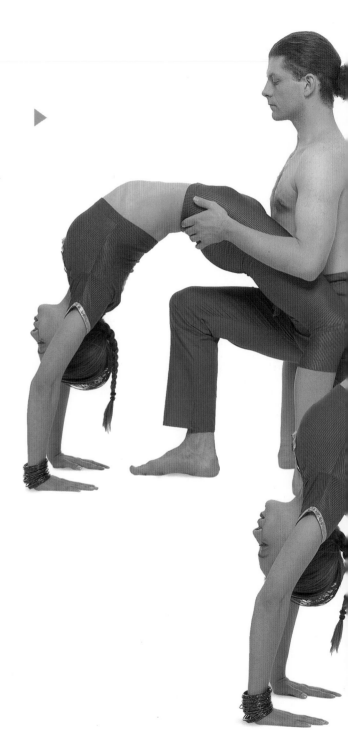

82

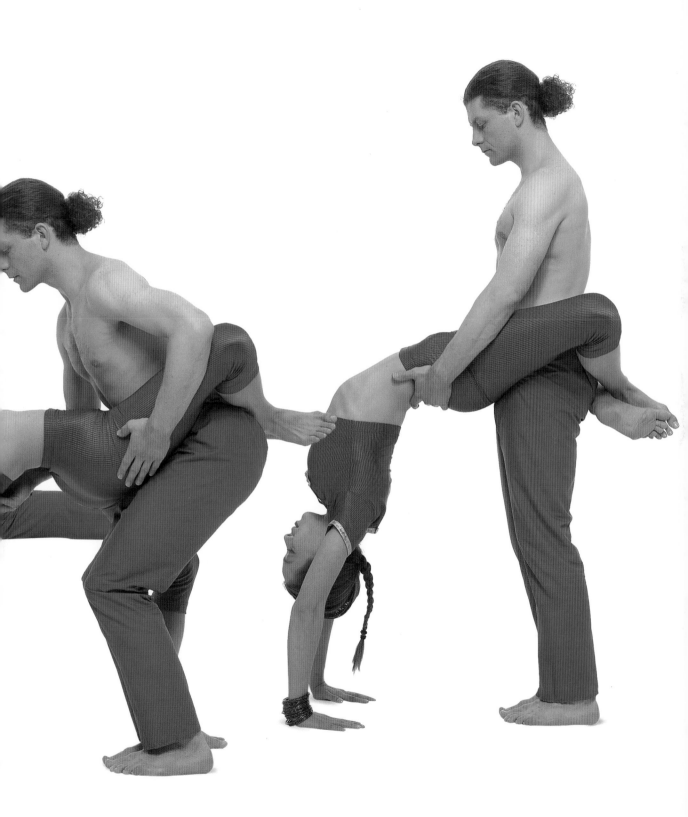

Splits

'You cannot give love unless you develop
your own capacity to love. Learn to flood
life with your love by giving love, asking
for nothing in return, expecting nothing,
wanting nothing. All glories may fade, die
away, or perish. The divinely sweet beauty
of love given, of tenderness shared, or
sympathy shown will always remain
untarnished. Adversity cannot dim its
brilliance nor age its beauty.'

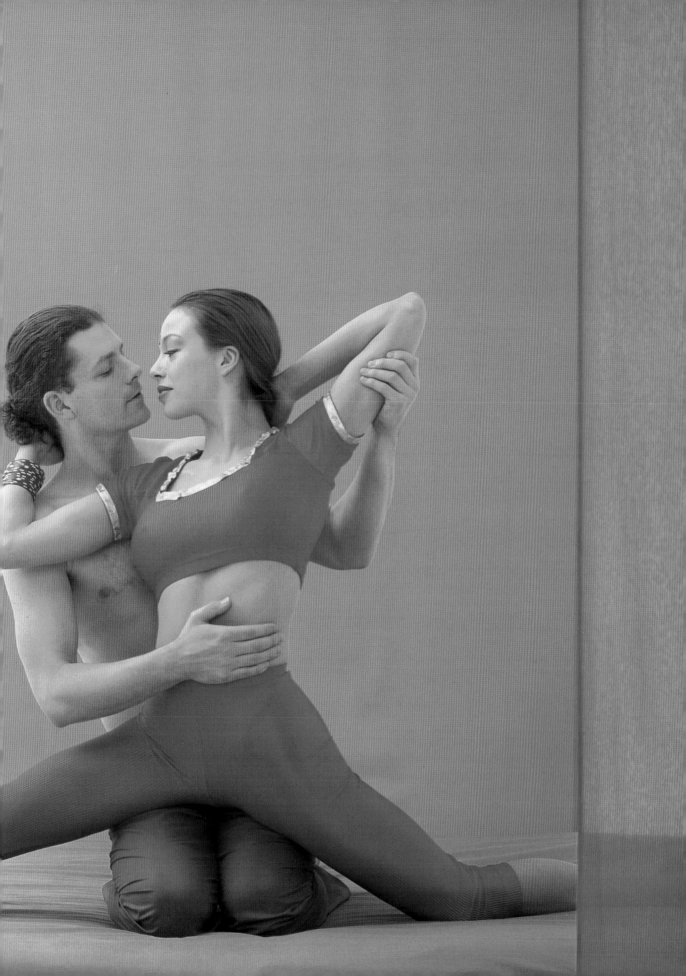

Splits Love Pose

This beautiful love pose is a perfect blend of a dancer's grace and poise combined with the flexibility of the hips and groin. To achieve this pose it is important for the woman to practise the Sitting Stretch (see page 30), Half Lotus Side Stretch (see page 60), the Warrior (see page 44) and Sitting Twist (see page 56) to release stiffness and help open up the hip area.

The man kneels down on the floor with his knees close together and his hips touching his heels, his feet flat down behind him. The woman half kneels down close to him on his left side so their bodies are touching and their arms caressing one another, she with her right arm around his right shoulder and her left arm on his right forearm and he with his left hand on her back and his right hand on her waist.

▸ She lunges her right leg over his thighs, creating a right angle to the floor, making sure that her lunge is deep enough so her knee does not extend over her foot. She balances on her left knee and her left hand moves to her waist, covering his hand. ▸ From this position she slides her right leg in a perfectly straight line and extends her left leg behind her until her weight is fully on his body. She points both her feet and balances between her right heel and left knee. She gently lifts her spine up toward her partner so her back is leaning on his chest, reaches her arms behind her and takes her right arm around the man's head in order to twist her body toward him so she can still gaze lovingly into his eyes.

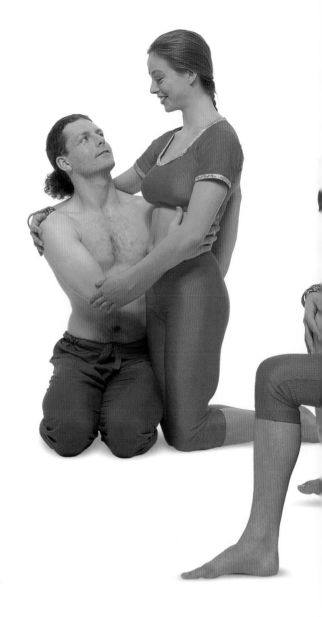

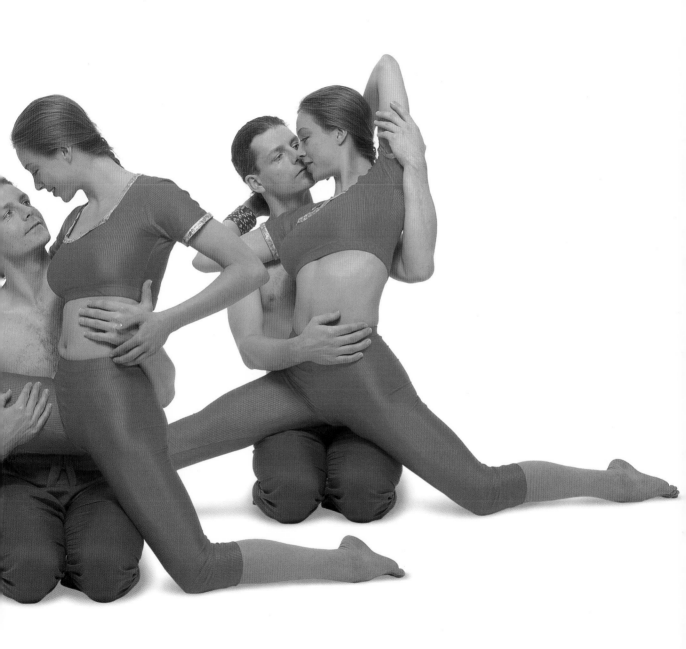

The Swan

'To give love is total freedom; to demand
love is pure slavery. The sun gives and
demands nothing. The earth, the moon, the
rains, the spring, the flowers, and the
rivers – everywhere in nature, and among
plants and animals, the universal rhythm is
to give lovingly and not to demand love
from others. We must open our hearts and
give willingly, openly, and without motive.'

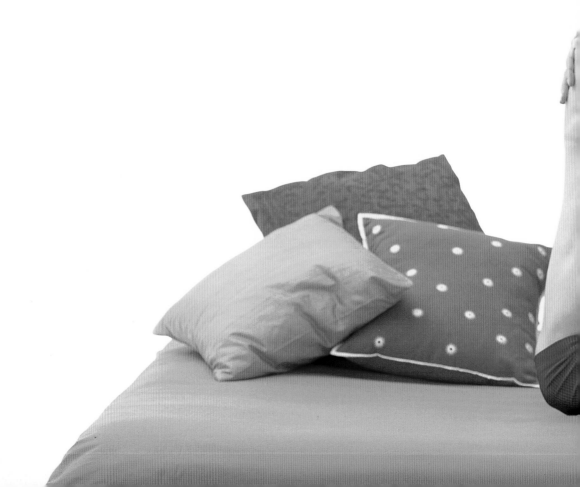

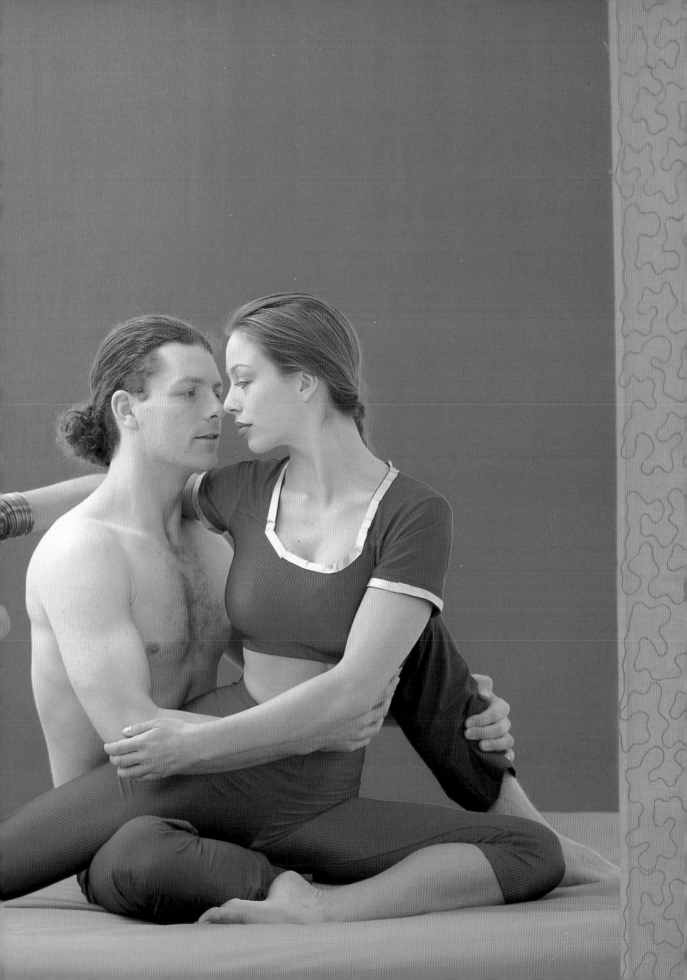

The Swan Love Pose

In order to achieve this love pose it is important for the woman to practise the Cobra and Bow (see page 28), the Standing Bow (see page 40) and the Locust (see page 54) in order to improve the strength and flexibility of her lower back and the Sitting Twist (see page 56) to help rotate her spine easily. Some people might find the final position too difficult to achieve and if this is so can finish with position 2 instead.

The couple begin the pose sitting down on the floor or a divan holding each other in a loving manner. The woman sits in front of the man, leaning on her left buttock with both legs tucked under so her knees and feet are together. She leans on the man and turns her back toward him so her right cheek caresses the left side of his face. He sits upright with his left leg up in a 90-degree angle to the floor in line with his left hip and his right leg folded directly in front of him. He holds the woman firmly and she gently holds his hands. ▶ She lifts herself up on both knees and slides her body on to his right thigh. She extends her right leg behind her as far as possible while balancing her weight between her left leg and her partner's upper thigh. He drops his right hand to the floor and straightens his elbow in order to support her weight. She turns her back so she can face him and puts her right hand behind his head. ▶ She reaches behind his back and lifts her right foot up and arches her spine. She holds on to her foot and twists her body closer to his body. He takes his left hand to his left leg and kisses her gently on the mouth.

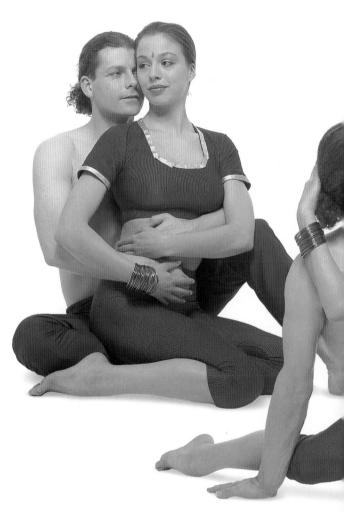

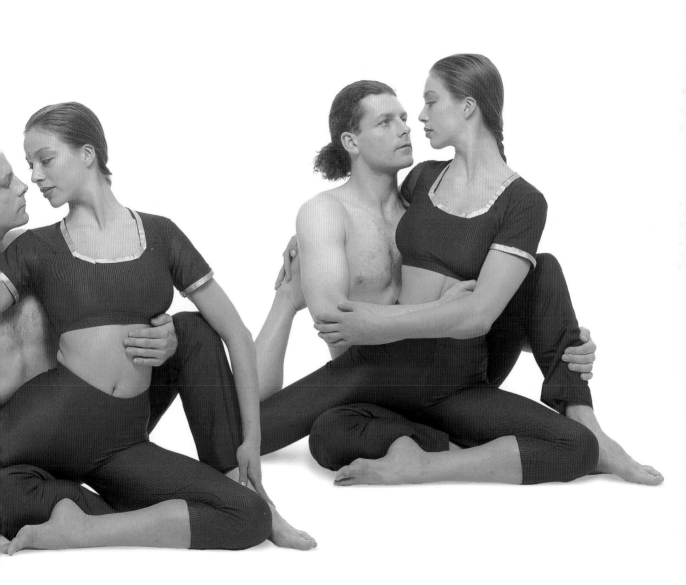

Half-Standing

'When the gates of heaven open and cosmic energy swirls in every fiber of being the two lovers reawaken their souls to the divine truth and beauty of everlasting love. They bask in the warmth of the sun's rays, knowing the stillness and pleasure of lasting joy and happiness and peace within.'

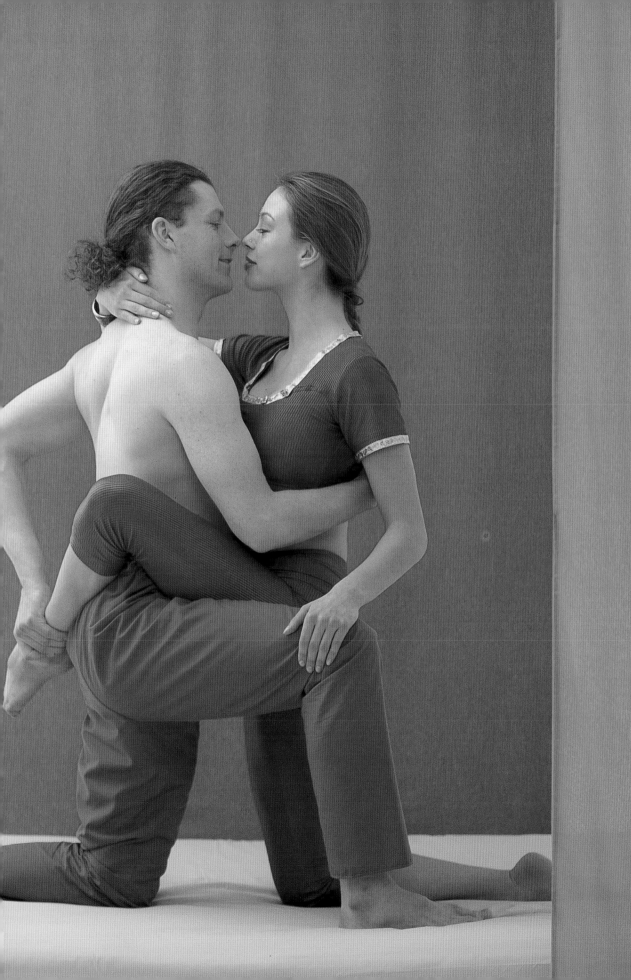

Half-Standing Love Pose

People who are relatively fit can achieve this pose without too much difficulty. Because of its simplicity it allows the intimacy of the couple to flourish as well as heightening sexual desire. The couple can enjoy the sex act mutually without added complications and can balance their weight equally between them.

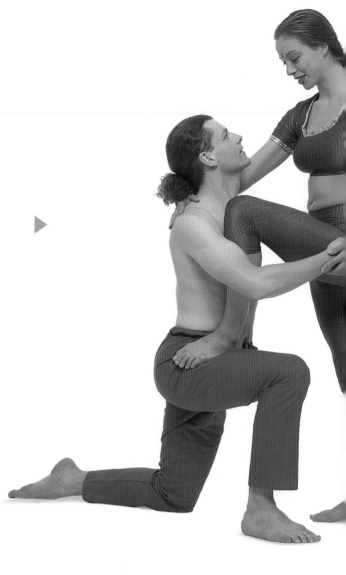

The couple begin by standing facing each other. The man drops to his left knee and keeps the right knee up with his foot firmly placed on the floor in a right angle to the floor. The woman lifts her left leg up and places her left foot on his right hipbone with her toes facing outward and her heel next to his groin. Her standing leg remains straight. She takes her right arm around his left shoulder and he takes his right hand to her left buttock. She gazes down at him and holds his right hand gently. ▶ She steps over his right thigh with her left leg and lowers herself down to his pelvis so her weight is resting on his body. Her left foot is firmly placed on the floor and her right leg is bent in order to distribute her weight evenly and allow movement between them. He grips her tightly around her waist and draws her closely toward him. She puts her left hand on his right knee to support her balance and pulls herself closer to him. ▶ She drops down to her right knee and curves her left leg around his waist so their bodies are directly touching. She points her toes and he takes hold of her foot with his left hand. He draws her body even closer as they gaze directly into each other's eyes.

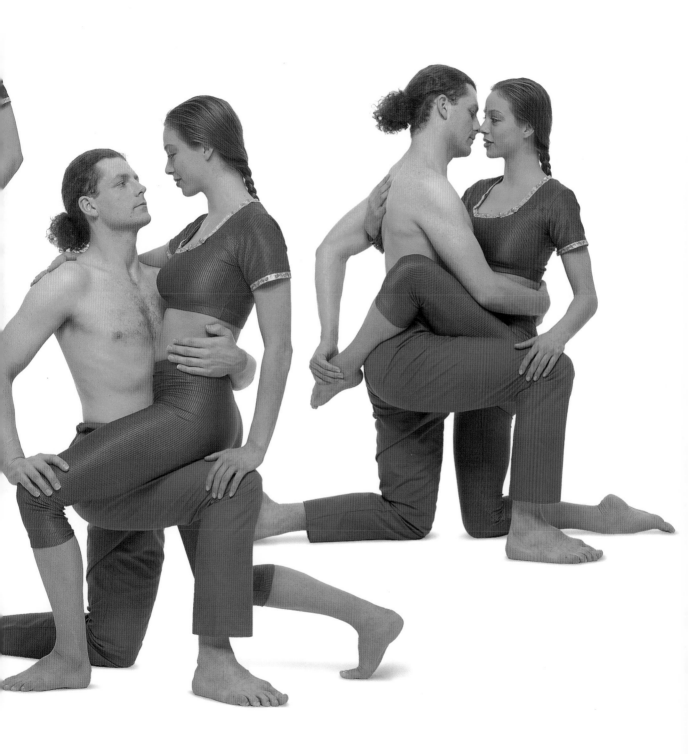

Table Top

'His dynamic love floods forth from his heart, breaks down all the barriers of his lover's heart and seeks and discovers a blissful fusion of oneness. The lover ennobles the beloved and yet retains his own individuality in all aspects of the love union. In such a blessed relationship the two become one and one never dominates or is deemed a victim of the other. This is the perfect splendor of true love.'

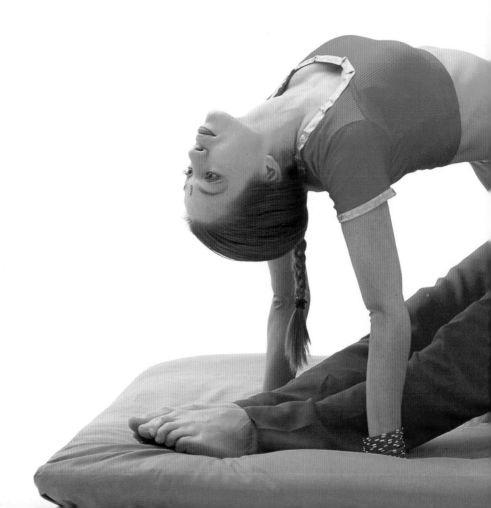

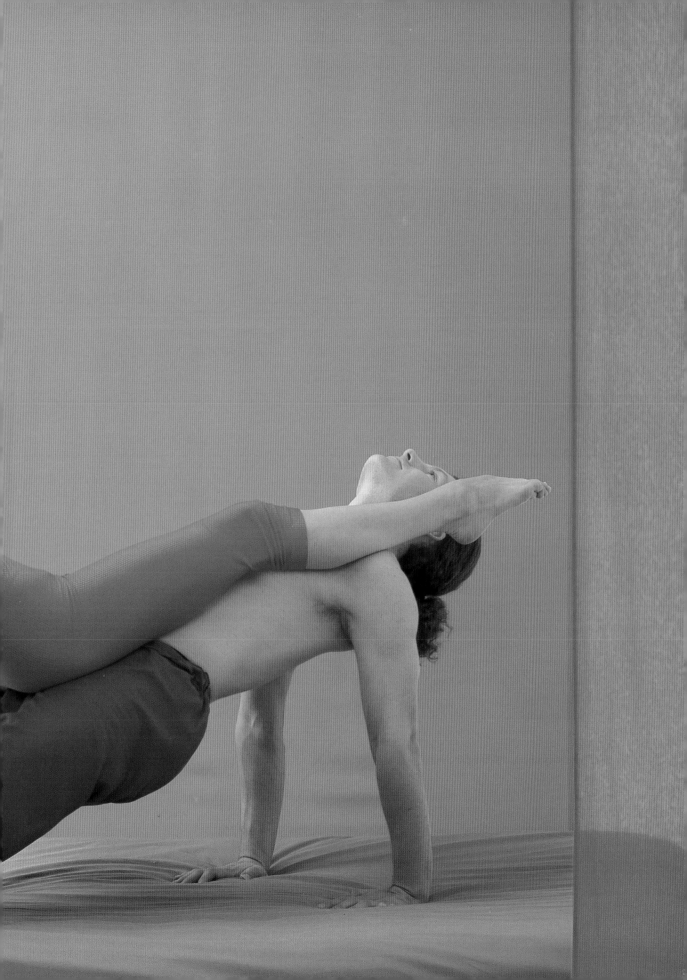

Table Top Love Pose

Only the practice of yoga asanas on a regular basis can prepare you to perform this love pose skilfully and correctly. It needs tremendous strength and stamina as well as flexibility by both partners to achieve the grace and beauty of this sensuous act.

The pose begins very simply with the couple in a loving embrace. The man is sitting up tall with his legs outstretched in front of him. The woman is sitting astride him with her knees on either side of his thighs. He is gently holding her upper back and she is holding him around his lower back. ▸ The woman leans back on the man's groin and places her hands down to the floor in preparation for the lift. Her elbows are straight and her fingertips facing the man. She raises her left leg over his right shoulder and keeps her spine in a straight line. The man supports her waist and points his feet down to the floor. ▸ The man takes his hands from the woman's back and places his palms on the floor in a direct line to his shoulders, fingertips pointing in line with the direction of his head. As he raises his hips as much as possible the woman is lifted automatically. She extends her body fully over his and leans backward, dropping her head back. Her left foot is pointed over his shoulder and her right foot drops to the floor to support her weight. Depending on her height, she may only be able to balance on her toes. The man supports his weight evenly between his heels and hands and lifts his hips up so his spine is in an exact straight line from his feet to his head.

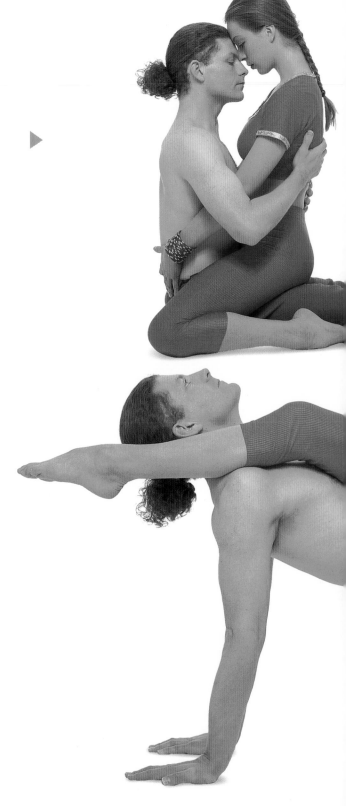

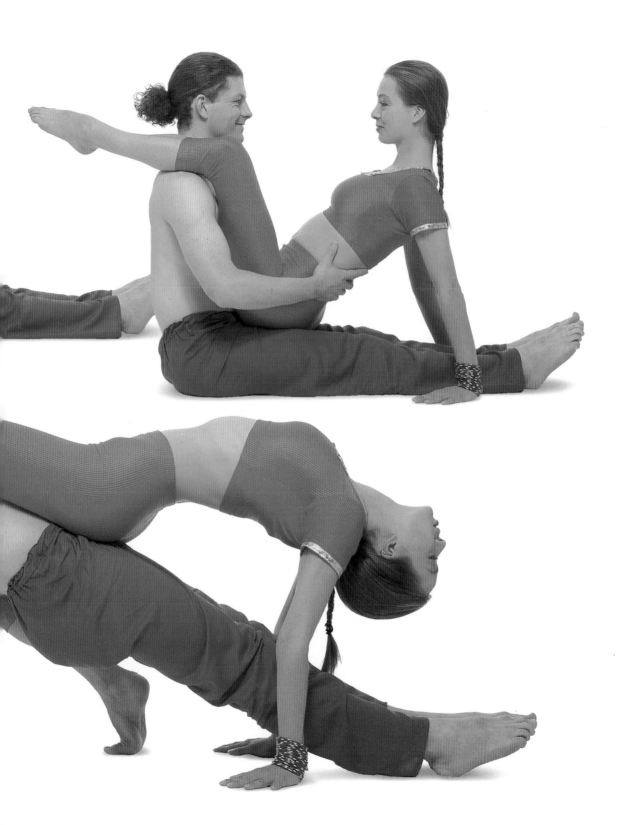

Leg Hook

'The purpose of human life is to blossom
like a flower with joy and love everlasting,
emitting fragrance and sweetness all
around. He who keeps his soul in tune with
the cosmic energy is like a flower which
has roots in the earth but looks up to the
heavens for sustenance. May the lovers
blossom together and permeate the
universe with divine scent.'

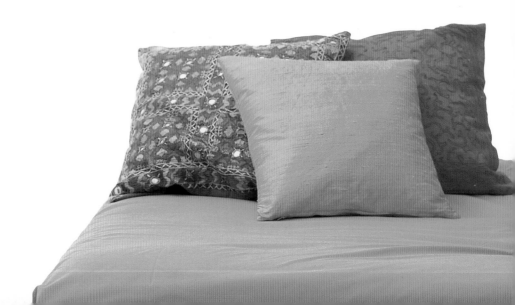

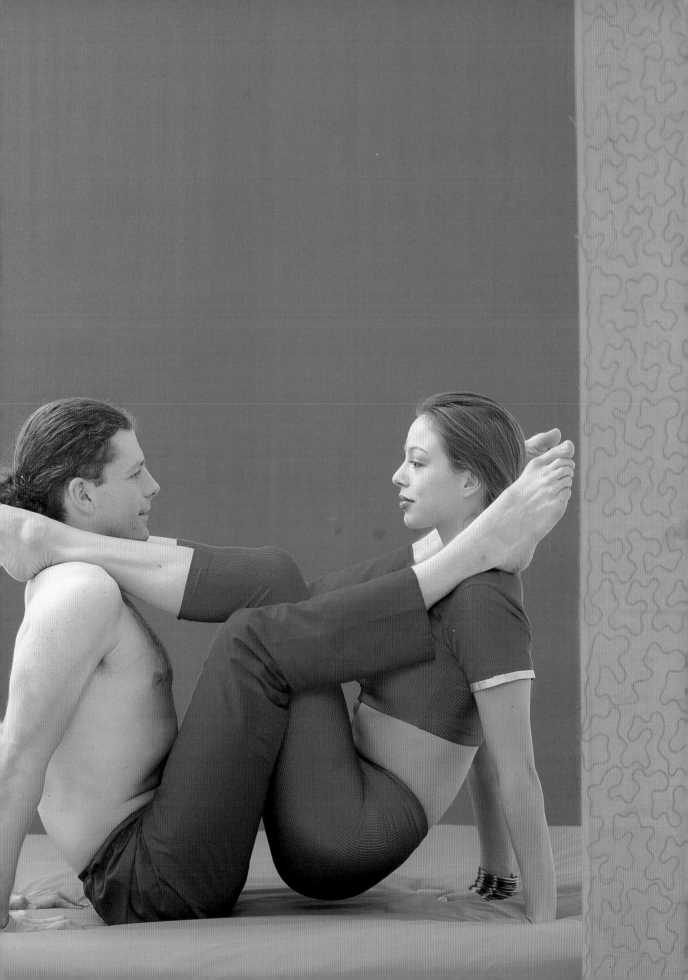

Leg Hook Love Pose

This erotic love pose unites the couple with equal passion and is relatively simple to perform. Both partners need to have a similar amount of strength in their arms and legs as well as in their pelvic and abdominal muscles. The Pelvic Stretch (see page 24) is a good exercise to help strengthen these muscle groups and the Dog Pose (see page 42) is particularly useful for building stamina and straightening the arms and legs.

To begin this pose the man sits erect on the floor with his knees facing outward and the soles of his feet together. The woman sits on top of the man with her feet also placed soles together. Their arms are gently wrapped around each other, his at her lower back and hers around the middle of his back.
▸ The woman leans back and places both her hands to the floor with her fingers pointing to the man. She straightens her arms in order to support her weight, lifts both legs up off the floor and places them on either side of her partner's head to rest on his shoulders. Both legs are exactly parallel and she is slightly off the ground, balancing on her hands. He moves his hands to her upper back to prepare to lift her and gazes directly into her eyes. ▸ Pushing down on her palms, she extends her elbows and lifts her body off the floor. When she is perfectly steady and balanced the man lifts his legs over her shoulders around her neck and places his hands behind him in order be able to free his hips and give himself extra support. The heads of the man and woman are at the same level to allow freedom of movement.

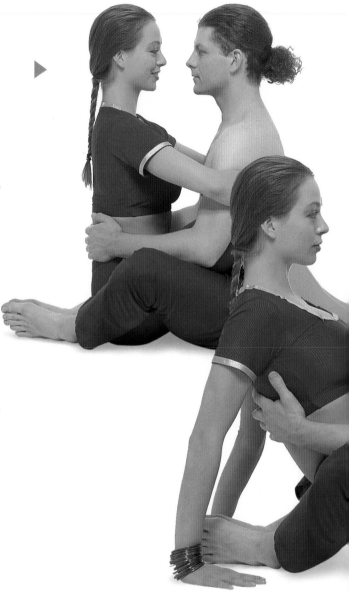

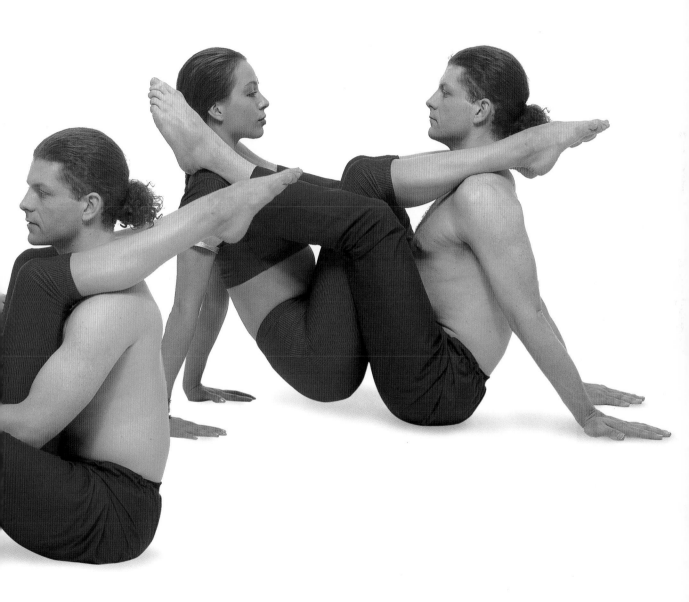

The Bow

'There is a universal demand in the heart
of man to seek his identity with all others
around him through love. In some it is an
urgent, conscious desire; in many others it
is a slow, unconscious need. But this urge,
to seek one's fusion with others through
love, is natural and irresistible to all.
We must always satisfy this urge and
continue for eternity to seek and find true
love. Only then will we find peace and
stillness within.'

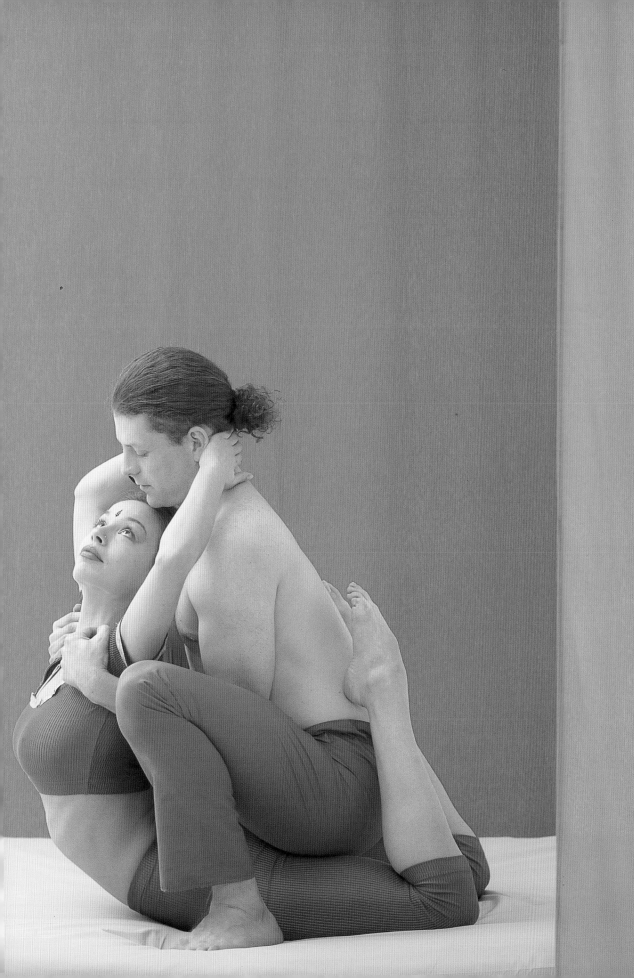

The Bow Love Pose

The Leg Stretch (see page 58), Back Arch (see page 62), Camel (see page 52), and Standing Bow (see page 40) are all excellent postures to practise when you wish to perfom this love pose. A strong back is required as well as a flexible spine to achieve the final position.

The woman begins by lying flat down on her stomach and the man stands up with his legs apart on either side of her hips. She lifts both legs up behind her while the man squats down on top of her. She lifts her back up, keeping her hips down, and supports her weight with her hands and elbows remaining on the floor. The man takes both hands under her armpits in preparation for the lift. ▶ She lifts her body all the way up into the classic Bow Pose (see page 28) and holds on to her ankles in a perfect arch. The man supports her by holding firmly on to her shoulders. ▶ She releases her legs and slides them down the man's back. She takes her arms around the back of his head and draws him closer to her.

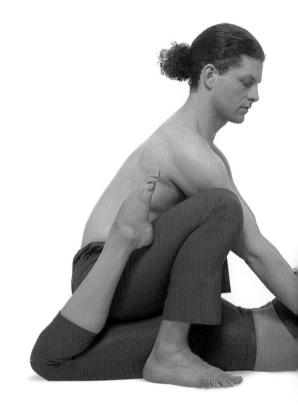

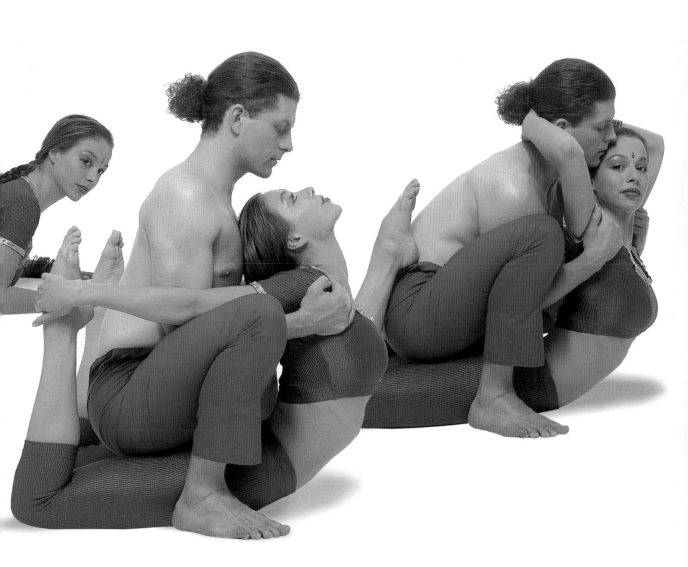

The Camel

'Without dedication and love, man is like an empty shell that crumbles into dust. Love transforms man's selfishness and self-centeredness into self-sacrifice. He who has not known love nor seen the beloved soul is like a guest entering an empty house. He departs disappointed, there being no spark or joy to encourage him to stay.'

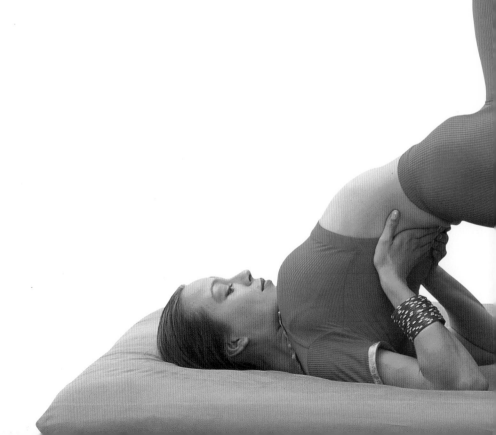

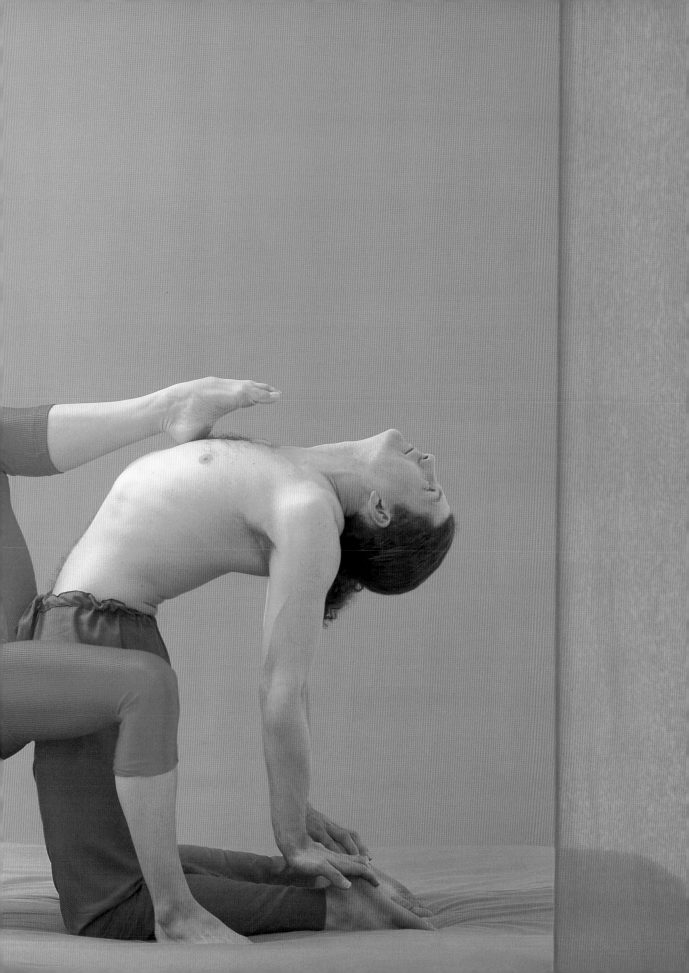

The Camel Love Pose

This Love Pose is physically demanding and both partners have to sustain their own position and not rely on each other for support. The Pelvic Stretch (see page 24), Camel (see page 52), Leg Stretch (see page 58) and Back Arch (see page 62) are good exercises for improving flexibility of the spine and building strength.

The man kneels down, knees and feet together. The woman sits on his thighs and wraps her legs around his waist. She places the soles of her feet together and gently holds the man around his shoulders. He holds her upper back and caresses her softly. ▶ The woman slides on to her back to the floor and lifts her legs up so her feet are in line with her hips. She slowly raises her pelvis as high as possible and arches her body so she is balancing on her shoulders and upper back. Her chin is locked into her chest. The man helps her by supporting her pelvis with his hands. She places her hands over his in a loving gesture. ▶ The woman takes her hands to the small of her back to support her weight. She tightens her buttocks and raises her hips even higher. At the same time, the man pushes his hips forward and stretches backward. His hips are in a direct line with his knees. He relaxes back as far as possible, tightening his buttocks while pushing his pelvis up to the woman. He opens his chest, holds on to his heels and drops his head down to relax his neck and throat while he thrusts forward. She raises her right leg off the floor and places her right foot on the middle of his chest.

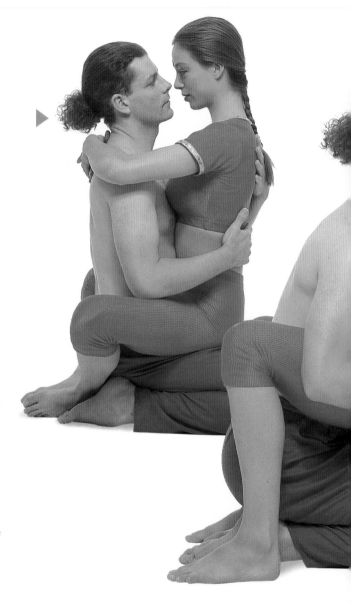

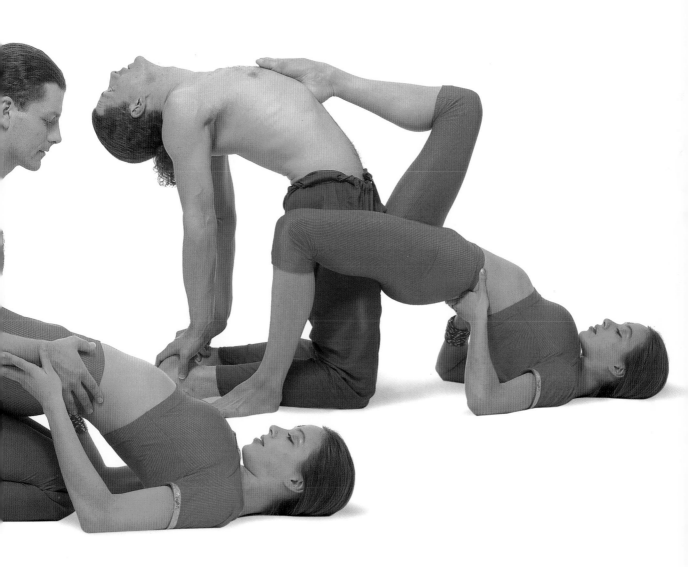

Side

'Love and devotion give man a purpose, a meaning and value to his existence. Love cannot protect life from death, but it can and will fulfill life's purpose. While death can bring life to an end it cannot undo the fulfillment of life's pleasures and joys. Every human being should gain this self-realization in order to transcend even the darkest thought into the light.'

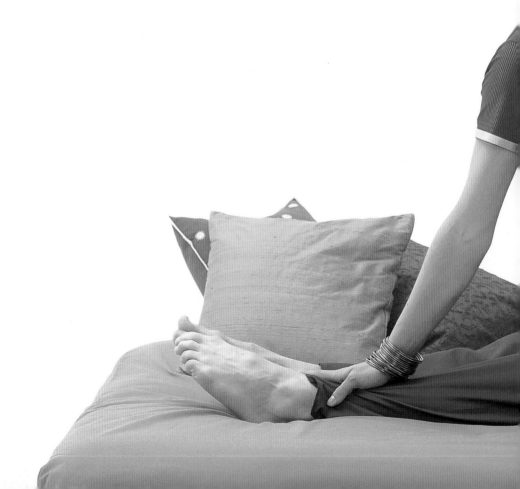

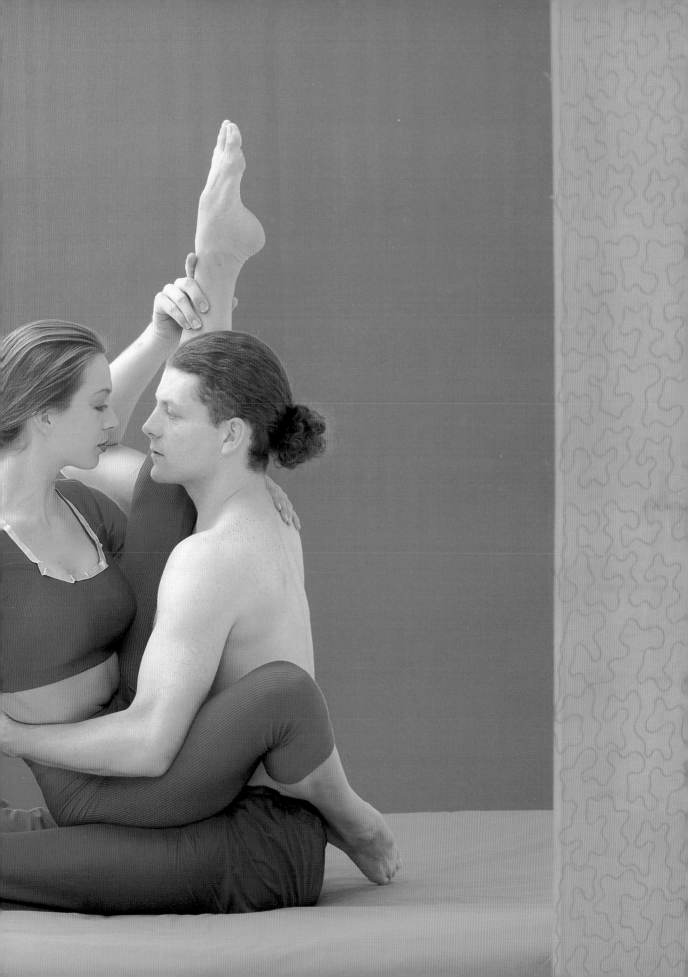

Side Love Pose

The beauty of this pose lies in its simplicity and truth. As the pose requires little movement it is a perfect opportunity for the couple to connect with each other's energy flow. In the Heart Chakra pose (see page 64) the energy contact flows through the chakras to unite at the level of the crown. Meditate on this thought and feel as if you are uniting sexually to connect with the universal cosmic flow of energy. Keep the eye contact constant and you will have a feeling of floating into divine bliss.

The man begins this pose by sitting comfortably on the floor, his legs outstretched in front of him and his spine erect. The woman sits sideways on the left side of his lap so her legs and feet are together alongside his right hip. The man takes his arms lovingly around her hips and the woman places her arms around his shoulders. They gaze deeply into each other's eyes. ▶ The woman leans back and places her left hand on the floor to support her weight. She bends her left leg and wraps it tightly around the man's waist. She lifts her right leg and points her foot over his left shoulder so her leg is in a straight line. The man takes his right palm to the floor to support the change in the woman's movement. They are still looking directly at each other. ▶ With his right arm, the man grasps the middle of the woman's back to draw her closer. She places her left foot on the floor to support her weight and give her freedom to move. She takes her right arm around his shoulder so she can grip on to his body and points her toe harder to straighten her knee. They continue to gaze lovingly at one another.

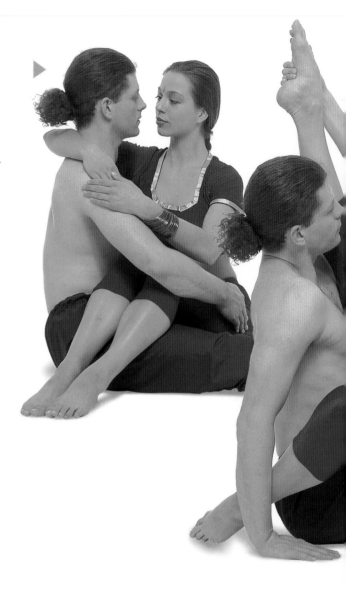

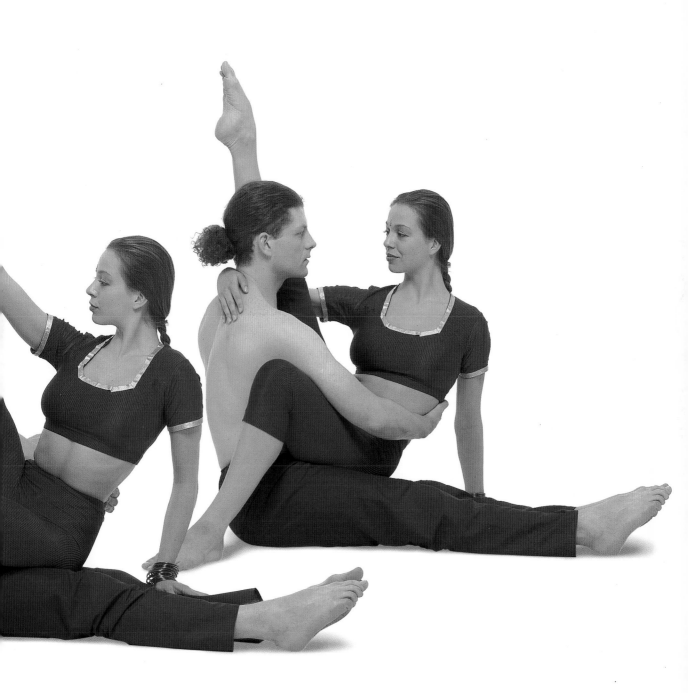

Half
Plough

'When our senses of love from our minds
and our bodies merge together there is a
quality of respect, a reverence that we feel
for each other. Respect of the intellect, of
thoughts and emotions, of dreams and
wishes, is foremost in promoting a loving
relationship. When total integration exists
between the mind, body, and soul we can
understand with true clarity the meaning
and importance of true love.'

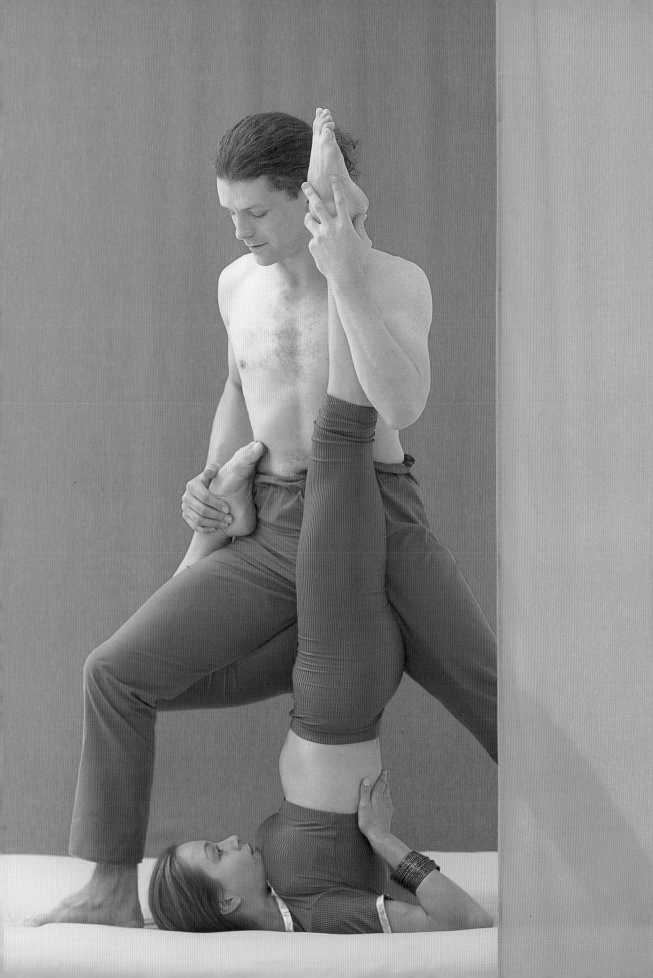

Half Plough Love Pose

This pose combines the classic Shoulder Stand described in the Plough (see page 48) for the woman and the Warrior pose (see page 44) for the man. The pose is dramatic in feeling and looks as if the man is dominating the woman. In reality it is a beautiful exchange of energy that is both erotic and sensuous.

The woman begins by lying flat on the floor, legs together and arms at her sides. She bends her knees to her chest, places her hands in the small of the back to support her spine and rolls back into an inverted position so her knees are on the top of her forehead. (If the abdominal muscles are weak she can place her hands on the floor to push herself back and then replace the hands on her lower back.) She lifts both legs up so her spine is as straight as possible, points her feet and locks her chin into her chest. The man stands close and pushes his weight under her hips to help straighten her spine even further. He holds her upper thigh with his right hand and both ankles with his left hand. ▶ The woman lowers her right leg to the floor directly behind her head, pointing her foot to extend her leg in a straight line. The man checks her position to make sure that she is in a 90-degree angle to the floor. ▶ When he is confident that her position is correct he lunges his left leg over her groin in front of her right leg and lowers himself. His left hand moves down to her inner thigh and his right hand holds on to her left ankle. He is at a perfect angle to look into her eyes.

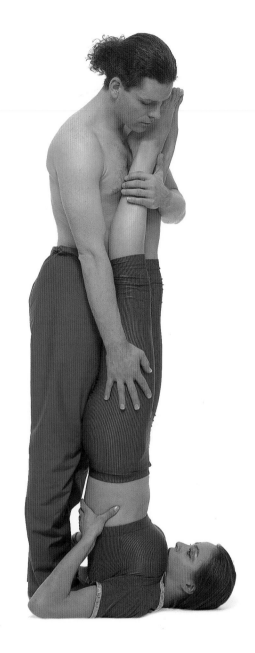

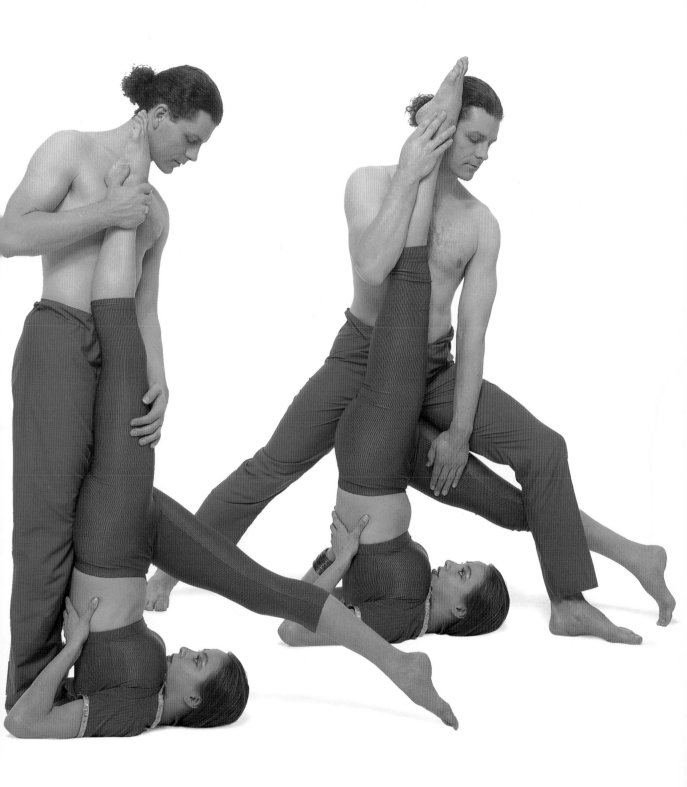

Salute to the Sun

'Love when it is pure has a revitalizing effect upon others, and in the presence of a truly loving person others grow and expand into a healthier state of being. Without deep reverence for the beloved such a refreshing stream of love cannot flow from the heart of the lover. The lovers must see one another with total objectivity without interfering with the personality. They encourage each other to grow, to unfold in the blinding light of the sun's power and strength.'

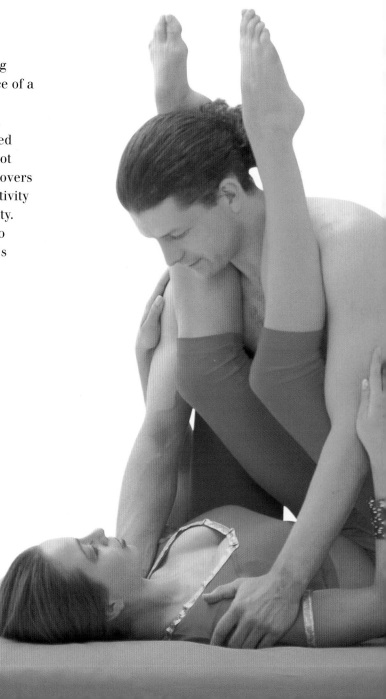

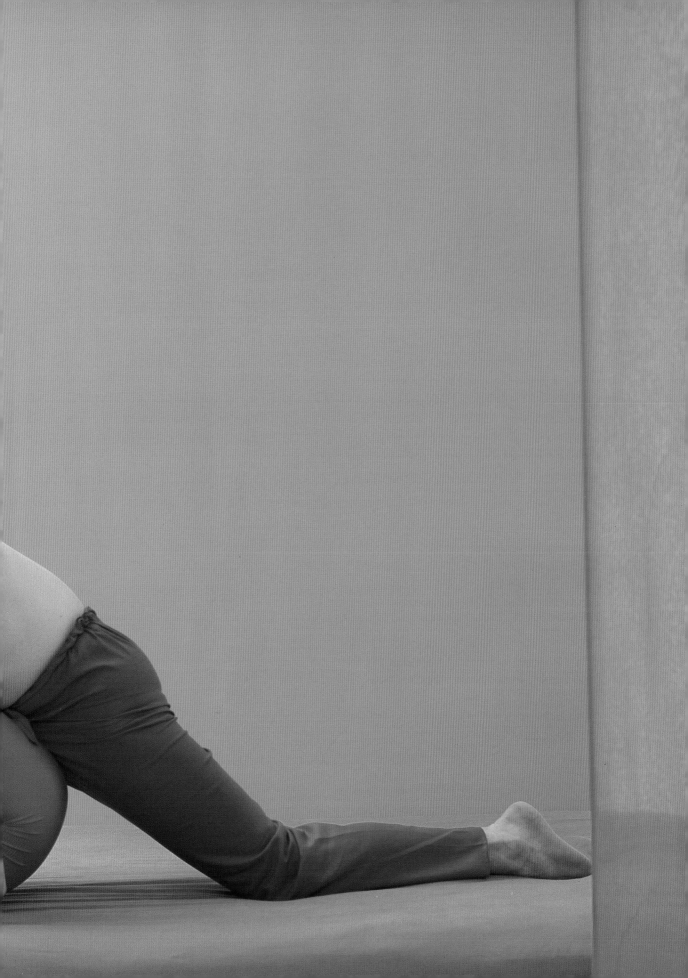

Salute to the Sun Love Pose

This pose is a series of flowing movements that require muscular strength on the part of the man and extreme flexibility in the woman. All the exercises in this book will help you reach a fitness level so you can achieve this pose with greater ease and confidence. The Head to the Knee (see page 50) and Half Lotus Side Stretch (see page 60) are excellent ways to improve flexibility, while the Warm Up (see pages 18–21) and the Balance (see page 22) are good for developing physical strength.

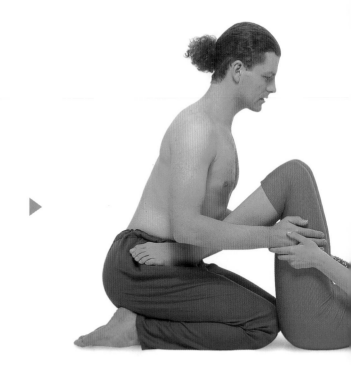

The man begins by kneeling in front of the woman. His knees are together and his feet are under his hips. The woman lies on her back facing him. Her legs are lifted up and her feet placed on either side of his hipbones with her toes pointing outward. They hold on to each other's hands. ▶ The man places his hands on the floor on either side of the woman's body and simultaneously the woman brings her knees to her chest and begins to roll back. The man jumps back into a full leg extension and balances on his toes while the woman continues to roll back, legs together and toes pointed. The man's chest and groin are pressing against the woman; she is holding her feet. ▶ The woman bends her knees, opens her legs and places each leg on the man's shoulders. She keeps both legs parallel and her toes pointed. He drops his left knee to the floor as he lunges forward with his right leg, his foot close to her left hip. She holds his upper arms and he holds her shoulders.

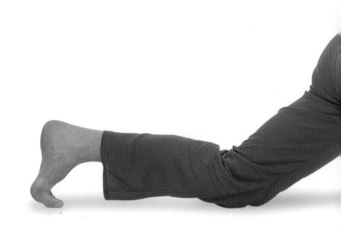

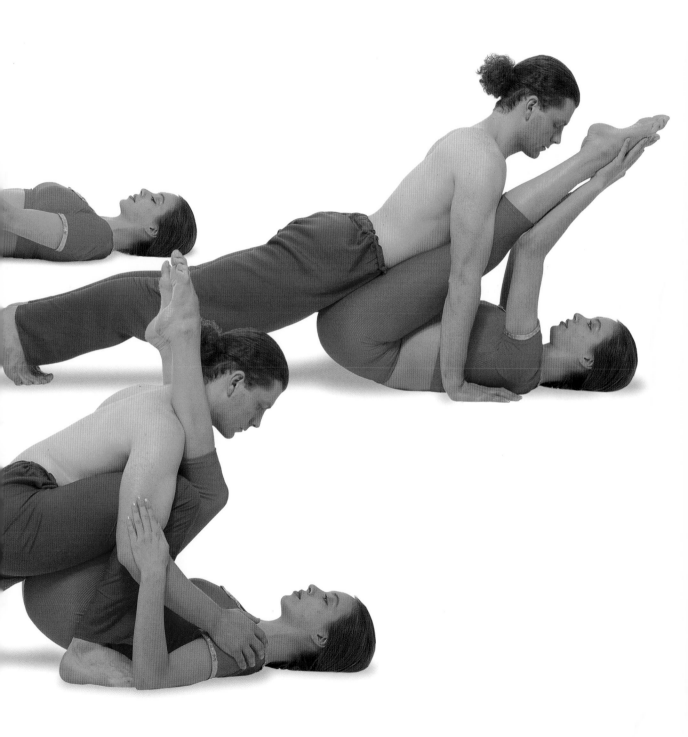

Diagonal Repose

'He who constantly throws around him a vibrant light of wondrous enchantment, himself forming an island of peace and contentment in the stormy life of uncontrollable fears, is a blessed man. He who seeks the Divine Love and Light will smash dark shadows and confusions all around him. He will truly live a spiritual life full of truth, harmony, and beauty and obtain the essence of true love.'

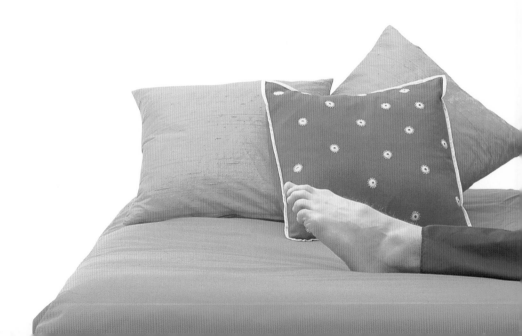

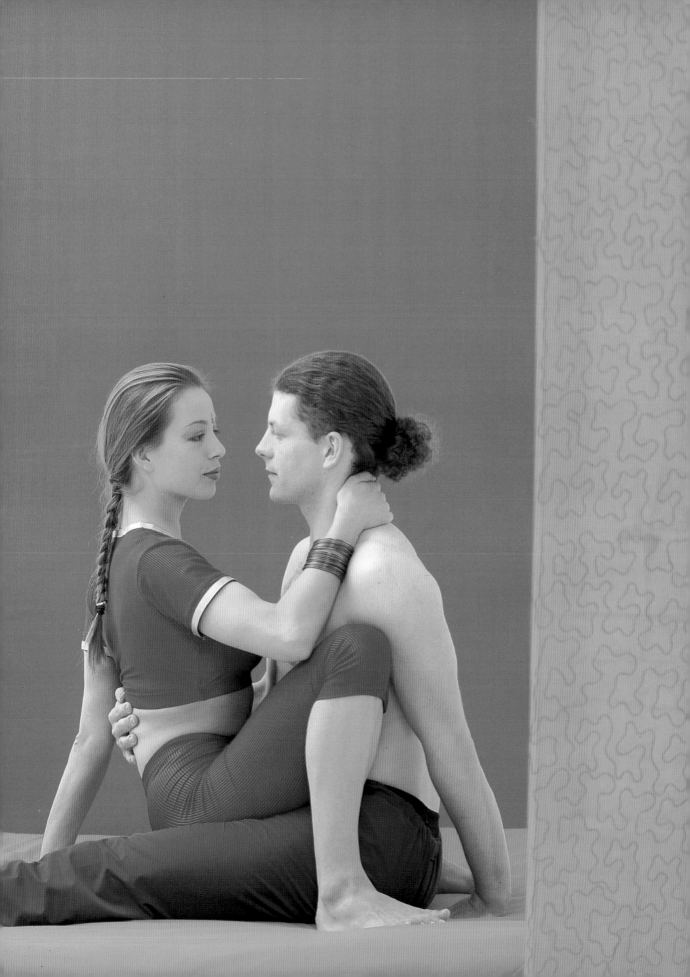

Diagonal Repose

This is a totally relaxed pose when the couple can enjoy the pleasure of lying together in a quiet manner. A repose rather than an active movement, it provides a pleasant way to end lovemaking. It is a subtle twist and the Sitting Twist (see page 56) is a good exercise to teach the fundamental benefit of twisting the spine.

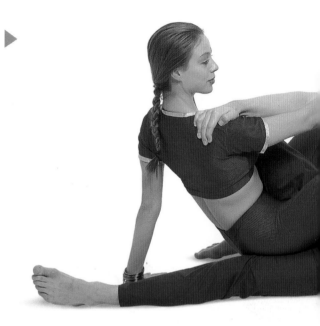

The man sits erect, legs outstretched in front of him. He brings his right knee up and positions it level with his left knee. He places his left hand behind him, fingers pointing toward his body, to support his weight and to help him lift his spine. The woman sits diagonally on top of him, her knees bent and her legs on either side of his hips. Her knees are up and her feet are firmly placed on the floor. She leans back and places her left hand on the floor behind her to support her weight. Her right hand moves to his left shoulder and his left hand to her right shoulder. Their arms are entwined as they look serenely into each other's eyes. ▸ At the same time the couple begin to lean backward toward the floor, holding gently on to each other's arms. The woman slowly extends both legs on either side of the man's waist and leans down on her left elbow. The man leans his body weight on his left elbow and extends his arm so he is holding the woman's upper arm. ▸ As they stretch down to the floor the couple gently twist their lower bodies toward each other and their upper bodies away. They are in a diagonal line with the woman facing one way and the man the other. She stretches both arms over her head and clasps her hands together with her palms facing outward, and he places both hands gently on her legs.

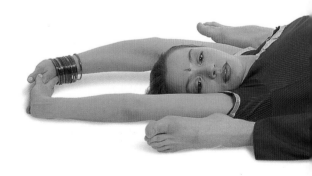

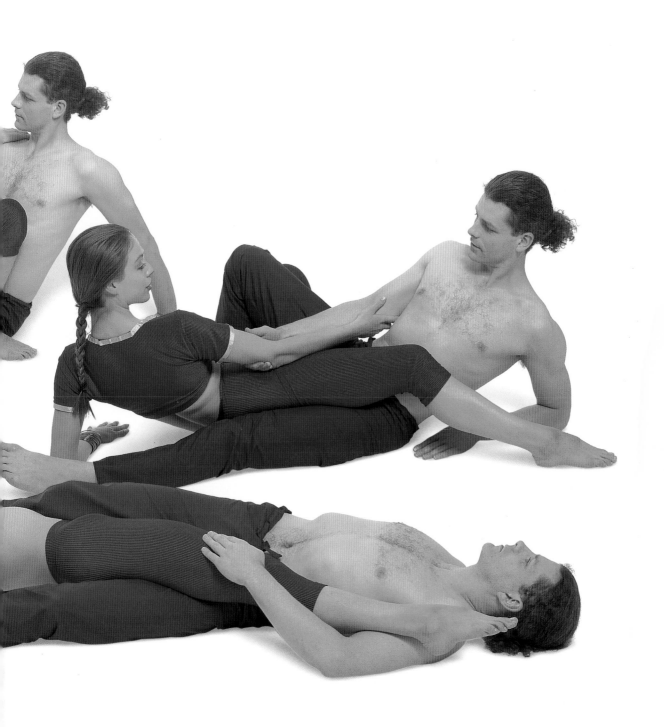

ACKNOWLEDGEMENTS

Publishing Director:
Laura Bamford

Commissioning Editor:
Jane McIntosh

Editor:
Diana Vowles

Assistant Editor:
Catharine Davey

Art Director:
Keith Martin

Senior Designer:
Ben Barrett

Designer:
Simon Balley

Photography:
Gary Houlder

Stylist:
Hannah Moseley

Hair and Make-up:
Esther Jones

Production Controller:
Dawn Mitchell

Sportswear kindly supplied by Sportique Fitness UK.
For catalogue of the full range of fitness wear,
phone 01773 608880.

Cushions kindly supplied by Neal Street East.